Surgical MCQs

To Pauline and Jean

Surgical MCQs

J. L. Craven
BSc MD FRCS
Consultant Surgeon, York District Hospital

J. S. P. Lumley
MB BS FRCS
Professor of Vascular Surgery and Honorary
Consultant in Surgery, St Bartholomew's Hospital,
London

SECOND EDITION

Churchill Livingstone
EDINBURGH LONDON MELBOURNE AND NEW YORK 1985

CHURCHILL LIVINGSTONE
Medical Division of Longman Group UK Limited

Distributed in the United States of America by Churchill
Livingstone Inc., 1560 Broadway, New York, N.Y. 10036,
and by associated companies, branches and
representatives throughout the world.

First edition 1976
Second edition 1985
   Reprinted 1987
   Reprinted 1989

ISBN 0 443 03052 9

British Library Cataloguing in Publication Data
Craven, J.L.
   Surgical MCQs.—2nd ed.
   1. Surgery—Problems, exercises, etc.
   I. Title   II. Lumley, J.S.P.
   617'.0076   RD37.2

Library of Congress Cataloging in Publication Data
Craven, J.L. (John Leonard)
   Surgical MCQ's.
   Rev. ed. of: Surgical MCQ's for undergraduates.
c1976.
   1. Surgery—Examinations, questions, etc.
I. Lumley, J. S. P. (John Stuart Penton) II. Craven,
J. L. (John Leonard).   Surgical MCQ's for undergraduates.
III. Title.   IV. Title: Surgical M.C.Q.'s. [DNLM:
1.   Surgery—examination questions.   WO 18 C898s]
RD37.2.C73 1985   617'.0076   84-12147

Produced by Longman Singapore Publishers Pte Ltd.
Printed in Singapore

Preface to the Second Edition

Revision of the text has allowed us to delete or modify those questions which we have found to have poor discriminant powers and to add some new questions which we hope will provide a more complete test for the undergraduate surgical student.

York and   J. L. C.
London, 1985   J. S. P. L.

Preface to the First Edition

An examination system which is to assess the results of a number of years of study should do so fairly, uniformly and reliably, it should cover as much of the syllabus as possible, and be able to differentiate between good and bad candidates in a consistent manner. The objective test succeeds to a large degree in fulfilling these requirements but in itself it must not be a handicap to the candidate who should be well versed in this form of examination technique.

It is not claimed that the questions in the subsequent chapters will provide a painless method of passing the undergraduate's surgical finals, for it is hoped that the horizon of examining boards will include data obtained from other important spheres such as continuous assessment, long term case studies, oral assessment and conventional essay-style questions. It is hoped that the book will provide the student with an introduction to objective testing and, in particular, with a method of both testing and improving his surgical knowledge.

We are grateful to Churchill Livingstone for the speedy and effective help they gave us in publishing this book.

April, 1976   J. L. Craven
J. S. P. Lumley

Introduction

Objective Testing

The perfect examination would be one in which the student was accurately assessed in his knowledge, comprehension, application, analysis and evaluation of material pertinent to the subject being examined. The use of the essay type question paper as the sole means of assessment has been criticised because of its reliance on subjective (and therefore unmeasurable) qualities.

For several years educationalists of many different disciplines have sought methods of objective testing which examined all the above mentioned qualities. In all objective tests the student has to choose the correct response out of one or more alternatives, his answers being either right or wrong. The subjective judgement of the examiner thus plays no part in this form of examination. Objective testing has been used extensively in the USA since the end of the Second World War, but introduction in the UK has been slow, and it has reached the universities generally via schools and technical colleges. However, a multiple choice question paper is now in use in most medical schools and it has been necessary for both the medical student and his teacher to become fully acquainted with the uses and abuses of this testing technique. It is appropriate here to consider the merits of the various examination techniques and, perhaps most important, to compare objective testing with the traditional essay question.

The Essay

Students and examiners have questioned the effectiveness of an essay paper in measuring the attainment of a number of years of study. The area covered by such an examination is very limited, the more so when a wide choice of questions is allowed. It thus encourages the students to 'spot questions' and to concentrate on only part of the syllabus. The marking of essays is time consuming and unreliable, there being marked variations in an individual examiner's reassessment of papers as well as between examiners. This variation makes comparison on a national level difficult and is further accentuated by what has been described as the deep psychological barrier of examiners to allocate more than seventy per cent of the total marks allowed for any given essay question. However the essay does determine the candidate's ability to write clear and legible English, it tests his ability to collect and quantitate material and it assesses his powers of logic, original thought and creativity. In terms of cost the essay question is cheap to produce but it is expensive to mark.

The Composition of Objective Questions

The objective form of examination is best composed by a panel of examiners, each having a complete understanding of the syllabus and a thorough knowledge of the field of study. The panel must first decide the parts of the syllabus to be covered by the examination, and the level of knowledge required by the candidate. The type of objective test and the number of options per question is decided and each member of the panel prepares a set of questions for the group to consider. A multiple choice question consists of a stem (the initial question) and four or more options; one of these options in the multiple choice question is correct and this is known as the key, the incorrect responses being known as the distractors. In the case of multiple response questions, there may be more than one correct response. (This form of question has also been termed multiple completion, multiple answer, multiple true or false and the indeterminate response by various authorities, but in most centres, and in this test, it will subsequently be referred to as a multiple choice question.)

Stem and options should be brief using the minimum number of words and the instructions should be clear and simple, the language used being appropriate to the verbal ability and requirement of the candidate. The questions must always be of some educational value. The words 'always' and 'never' should be avoided and the stem should preferably not be in the negative. There should be no recurrent phrase in the options which can be included in the stem. The key (the correct option or options) must be wholly correct and unambiguous. It is important for the correct response to be in different positions in each of a group of questions and some form of random allocation may be necessary. The distractors (the wrong options) are the most exacting and challenging part of objective question composition and the standard of an objective test is probably best assessed in terms of the quality of its distractors. They must always be plausible, yet completely wrong. They should be in a parallel style to the key and they should not contain clues. Common misconceptions form good distractors. 'None of them' or 'all of them' are not satisfactory distractors. Four options are thought by many authorities to be sufficient.

After the draft questions have been collected, it is advisable for a panel of examiners to assess their value and limitations. Inaccurate and irrelevant material is then excluded. Even the most experienced of examiners will find that a panel will offer constructive criticism on the majority of his questions. Ideally, once the panel has accepted a series of questions these should be pre-tested on a group of students and the results analysed. It is desirable for a question to have been pre-tested on 300 to 400 students before it comes into regular use in a qualifying examination. The difficulty of a questions can be determined by calculating the percentage of students giving the right answer, and its discriminatory value (the ratio of correct/incorrect responses) calculated in a manner which takes into account whether or not the better students obtained the correct response. The facility value (difficulty index) records the percentage of correct responses and compares it with the total number of candidates. Additional information on the mean range of distribution of the answers can also be obtained with a discriminatory index and a bi-serial correlation coefficient (relating the total candidate response to an option, with the results of the top 27 per cent and the bottom 27 per cent of the candidates to the same option). Figures for both the discriminatory index and the bi-serial correlation coefficient range from plus 1 to minus 1. Questions with factors of less than 0.20 should be rejected (unless a few difficult or easy questions are to be included). Values of 0.21 to 0.29 are of marginal discriminatory value. The values 0.30 to 0.39 show a reasonable discriminatory power of the option, whereas results greater than 0.44 indicate good discrimination by a question of the candidates under test. The effectiveness of the question is also measured in terms of the number of students attempting it — the value of a question certainly cannot be assessed if a large number of students leave it out. Computer readouts on a series of questions will also provide the ranking of students, the scatter of the results and a raw score (i.e. the number of correct less the number of incorrect results).

The pre-testing, though very time consuming, greatly adds to the validity and reliability of the objective test. Using the results of these tests the panel can rephrase unsatisfactory questions and compile the definitive examination paper. The time allowed in the pre-test is not limited but the students are asked to note the time taken to complete the test; the time required for the final version is thus arrived at. This time should allow at least 90 per cent of the candidates to complete the paper. It is usual to start an examination paper with a few easier questions (i.e with a low difficulty index) and similarly a few difficult questions can be included at the end. It has been found that a good (wide) range of results is obtained by setting a large number of questions with average discrimination rather than including a large number with high or low discriminatory indices. Testing of the questions should not stop after the pre-testing phase, the information gained from each subsequent examination should be used to continuously review all the question material.

Obviously a series of questions which have been pre-tested and shown to be satisfactory is of great value to the examiner. Such questions can be used repeatedly provided they have not been freely available to the student. Security is an important factor, particularly when the number of questions is small and does not cover the whole syllabus. For this reason it is advisable to have a large number of questions available. It is reasonable to assume that if a student is capable of memorising the correct responses to a large number of questions (even if these are known to him) he will also have a passable knowledge of the syllabus.

A satisfactory bank of questions takes three to five years to build. After this time the questions can be grouped into sections and, whenever an examination paper is required, questions can be chosen at random from each section. Continuous updating and revision of this material should be undertaken and new material added regularly. The history of each question in the bank should be recorded. Repetitive use of the questions over a number of years allows annual standards to be compared.

The Student's Approach To Objective Testing

Any student required to undertake an objective test for a qualifying examination or postgraduate examination should ensure he has some preliminary experience in this form of testing. It is essential for him to know and have sampled the style of questions used by his particular examining board.

In any objective test all the instructions provided must be carefully read and understood and the student's designated number marked in the appropriate section, otherwise a computer marking system will reject the paper—this will not impress the examining authority.

The type of objective test used in medical education does vary and some of these types have already been discussed. Whatever form the question takes in the objective test it is essential that the student starts on his first quick 'run' through the questions by filling in all the answers he knows to be correct. On this first 'run' he should also mark (on the paper) the questions where he is fully acquainted with the material but is unsure of the correct response. On the second 'run' all his attention can now be given to this group of questions, in which he should be able to make an informed guess. Experience has shown that his chances of being correct in this situation are above average. He should, as one examiner expresses it, 'play his hunches'. The questions which he does not understand are probably best left unanswered as at best he can only hope for a 50 per cent chance of a correct response on a random basis in the true/false situation, and only a 25 per cent chance of a correct response in a four-item multiple choice question. In multiple choice questions the marking is usually positive, a mark being given for a correct answer and none for an incorrect one. In multiple response questions (as in this text) a mark is given for each correct response, whether this be true or false, and usually a mark is subtracted for each incorrect response. Most examination systems have now abolished the use of a correction factor for guessing as this was found to have little effect on the ranking of the candidates, it has also been realised that informed guessing is in itself a useful discrimination.

Lack of time is not usually a problem in medical objective testing. Since these tests are of the 'power' rather than the 'speed' variety, i.e. knowledge rather than ability against the clock is being tested. Excessive time may be a disadvantage to the candidate as repeated reassessment of the answers may distract from the correct response rather than produce imporvement. In the multiple choice situation it has been found that one minute is usually necessary per question although more time is required to answer a question containing a number of distractors.

Transcribing 300 items from a question paper to an answer sheet (i.e. 60 questions each with 5 options) takes a minimum of 10 minutes and the habit of leaving such transcriptions to the end of an examination is best avoided since, if rushed, it may introduce unnecessary inaccuracies.

Etymological Hazards

The rarity of absolutes in medicine means that a large variety of adjectives and adverbs are commonly used in its description. These increase the difficulty of both setting and answering multiple choice questions. Although one can questions the desirability of assessing knowledge which is dependent on the 'strength of an adjective', these adjectives do form the language of present day medical practice. This factor is borne out by their frequent use in the questions and answers of the present text. Nevertheless, the examiner must avoid ambiguity and in addition his questions must not contain clues to the correct answer. Such terms as 'invariable', 'always', 'must', 'all', 'only', and 'never' should be avoided since they imply absolutes and are therefore likely to be wrong.

The terms 'may' and 'can' also give rise to ambiguity. In medicine almost anything 'may occur' and statements using this phrase are unlikely to be completely wrong. If these terms are used and the student is able to answer that the question 'certainly may' or 'certainly may not', he has little chance of being wrong. The term 'sometimes' comes into the same category.

The adjectives and adverbs 'common', 'usual', 'frequent' (commonly, usually, frequently), 'likely' and 'often' are an integral part of everyday medical language but their use in the 'multiple choice question may also lead to ambiguity. Their meanings are very similar yet their values depend largely on the context of the question. Expressed as incidences they may well range from 30 to 70 per cent. They may be considerably modified by the addition of 'quite', 'most', 'very' and 'extremely'. The examiner must be particularly careful of his choice of these terms. The 'majority' implies more than 50 per cent, whereas the 'vast majority' implies nearly 100 per cent.

The term 'typical' is a useful one for multiple choice questions. Its meaning implies 'that which is found in clinical practice'. 'Characteristic' implies a time honoured diagnostic feature and 'recognised' an accepted text book feature. Less explicit, and therefore less desirable, terminology includes 'most authorities agree', 'generally assumed', 'probable', 'though to be', 'all reports indicate' and 'has recently been reported'. Further vague terminology used in medical practice yet best avoided in the multiple choice situation include 'associated with', 'accompanied by', 'related to', 'linked with' and 'lend support to'.

On the negative side, 'uncommon', 'unusual', 'infrequent' (uncommonly, unusually, infrequently), 'unlikely' and 'rare' are all terms commonly used yet their use in the multiple choice situation must not give rise to ambiguity. As with their positive equivalents they are markedly influenced by the addition of such terms as 'most' and 'very'. The term 'significant' is best kept for its statistical use and the terms 'increased' and 'more' should be restricted to direct comparative situations.

The terms 'demand' and 'should' indicate the examiner's personal opinion and, although their inclusion is questionable, the student is still required to indicate whether he thinks the opinion is valid.

In conclusion, words used in multiple choice questions, although giving rise to apparent ambiguity, remain those in common use in medical practice; both the examiner and the student must be fully conversant with their meanings and disadvantages in order to avoid any confusion. It is hoped that the questions which follow will also help in this regard.

Contents

How to use this book

The text, consisting of questions and answers ('true or false'), is arranged throughout in such a way that all questions appear on left-hand pages and all answers on right-hand pages.

In use the student may conveniently cover the right-hand page with a blank sheet on which to jot down his answers for comparison.

1 Fluid and electrolyte balance

1 **The normal adult value for**
   A urine output is 1.5 litre/day
   B insensible water loss is 200 ml/day
   C potassium requirement is 150 mEq (150 mmol)/day
   D protein requirement is 70 g/day

2 **In a healthy 70 kg male the**
   A total body water measures approximately 40 litres
   B extracellular fluid volume measures approximately 8 litres
   C Plasma volume measures approximately 3.5 litres
   D 'third space' fluid measures approximately 1 litre

3 **The pH of the extracellular fluid**
   A is maintained in health between 7.4 and 7.6
   B is maintained entirely by the buffering system of the intra- and extracellular fluids
   C is increased in hypovolaemic shock
   D decreases abruptly after a cardiac arrest

4 **A low serum sodium level**
   A is commonly present in the early postoperative period
   B may cause stupor and fits
   C should be treated with isotonic saline infusions
   D is associated with an impaired ability to excrete water

1 A **True**   in a temperate climate.
  B **False**   insensible loss via skin and lungs ranges from 700 to
                 1000 ml/day and will be increased during fever and
                 high ambient temperatures.
  C **False**   potassium requirements of the healthy adult are 40 to
                 60 mEq (40 to 60 mmol)/day. There are excessive
                 losses during starvation, hypercatabolic states,
                 intestinal obstruction and diarrhoea.
  D **True**   this is increased in hypercatabolic states such as
                 burns and severe sepsis.

2 A **True**   the average values are 62 per cent of total body
                 weight in males and 52 per cent in females.
  B **False**   the extracellular fluid volume measures about 22 per
                 cent of the body weight, i.e. approximately 15 litres.
                 This includes plasma volume, lymph and interstitial
                 fluid.
  C **True**   the whole blood volume being approximately 5 litres.
  D **True**   this is the fluid normally in the pleural and peritoneal
                 cavities and the cerebrospinal fluid together with the
                 secretions in the alimentary tract. This component
                 enlarges considerably at the expense of the extra
                 cellular fluid volume in peritonitis, intestinal
                 obstruction and with any large inflammatory area.

3 A **False**   in the healthy individual the pH is maintained between
                 7.35 and 7.42.
  B **False**   by the buffering capacity of the bicarbonate/carbonic
                 acid system, the phosphate buffer system and the
                 buffering properties of the serum proteins and
                 haemoglobin. Additional regulation is by the lungs
                 and kidneys.
  C **False**   shock is always associated with a metabolic acidosis.
  D **True**   the absence of tissue perfusion results in a rapid fall in
                 the pH of the extracellular fluid.

4 A **True**   increased antidiuretic hormone production occurs
                 resulting in increased water retention.
  B **True**   this complication may be confused with a cere-
                 brovascular accident.
  C **False**   3 per cent (hypertonic) saline should be administered
  D **True**   in order to produce a diuresis and overcome the
                 inability of the kidney to excrete water in
                 hyponatraemia.

5   The sodium ion
   A is the principal regulator of the intracellular volume
   B is the major ionic component of the extracellular fluid volume
   C is present in greater concentration in intracellular fluid than extracellular fluid
   D is excreted in larger amounts than normal in the early postoperative period

6   Potassium deficiency should be suspected
   A in cases of paralytic ileus
   B when the patient's reflexes are exaggerated
   C if there is an increase in height and peaking of the T waves of an ECG
   D in alkalotic states

7   Potassium deficiency
   A can be effectively monitored by the serum potassium levels
   B may render digitalis therapy more dangerous
   C should be treated with an infusion of normal saline with potassium supplements
   D is not usually present in intestinal obstruction

8   The effects of a major extracellular fluid deficiency
   A include a decreased skin turgor
   B include hypotension
   C include excessive salivation
   D may be corrected by an infusion of isotonic saline

9   Extracellular fluid losses are often extensive in
   A intestinal obstruction
   B peritonitis
   C pancreatitis
   D hepatic coma

5 A **True**   because of the low intracellular concentration of
   B **True**   sodium, ionic movement of the ion into or out of the
                    extracellular fluid is accompanied by an immediate
                    movement of fluid into or out of the intracellular
                    space.
   C **False**   sodium is almost exclusively an extracellular ion.
   D **False**   there is an initial postoperative retention of sodium.

6 A **True**   potassium deficiency may be both a cause and an
                    effect of paralytic ileus. A diminished intracellular
                    potassium results in atony of both visceral and
                    skeletal muscle.
   B **False**   the reflexes are decreased.
   C **False**   the myocardium is also subject to muscle atony and
                    an ECG shows a prolongation of the Q–T interval,
                    depression of the ST segment and eventual inversion
                    of the T wave.
   D **True**   when there is excessive chloride loss, potassium
                    excretion rises as the kidney attempts to conserve
                    hydrogen ions.

7 A **False**   the major store of potassium is intracellular and the
                    serum levels may be normal in the presence of a large
                    intracellular deficit.
   B **True**   potassium deficiency enhances the effect of digitalis
                    and dysrhythmias are prone to occur
   C **True**   the infusion should not contain more than 40 mEq
                    (40 mmol) of potassium/litre and should usually not
                    be administered at more than 15 mEq (15 mmol)
                    potassium/hour.
   D **False**   a deficient intake and excessive losses of potassium
                    into the bowel lumen often lead to potassium
                    deficiency in this condition.

8 A **True**   due to the resultant hypovolaemia.
   B **True**
   C **False**   the mucous membranes are drier than normal.
   D **True**   this solution and other isotonic electrolyte-containing
                    fluids such as Ringer's lactate are the most effective
                    agents for restoring extracellular fluid.

9 A **True**   in all these conditions there may be extensive internal
   B **True**   translocations of fluid from the extracellular
                    compartment to the 'third space' (see Q.2).
   C **True**
   D **False**   in liver failure the extracellular fluid volume is usually
                    increased.

10   Excessive vomiting or loss of gastric secretion by nasogastric suction
   A   produces a metabolic alkalosis
   B   results in a low serum potassium
   C   may produce renal failure
   D   should be treated with isotonic saline infusions

11   Increases in the extracellular fluid volume can be accurately assessed and fluid overloading avoided by
   A   serum electrolyte determinations
   B   the measurement of the central venous pressure (CVP)
   C   the measurement of hourly urine volumes
   D   serial body weighing

12   Anuria in the postoperative period
   A   is defined as the production of less than 500 ml of urine/day
   B   should be treated with an initial 'waterload', i.e. a 4 litre fluid infusion
   C   is associated with hypernatraemia and dehydration
   D   is usually treated by renal dialysis

13   The anuric patient
   A   should have a fluid intake of 1 to 1.5 litres per day
   B   should have no potassium administered
   C   is at risk from metabolic alkalosis
   D   should be on continuous urinary catheter drainage

10 A **True**   there is an excessive loss of hydrogen and chloride
   B **True**   ions producing an alkalosis. As the loss of chloride
   C **True**   continues the kidney is unable to reabsorb the tubular
   D **True**   sodium and substitutes potassium in the tubular
                 urine. Thus potassium excretion rises and serum
                 potassium falls. The associated loss of fluid often
                 gives rise to uraemia. These metabolic upsets usually
                 respond to infusions of isotonic saline but
                 occasionally potassium needs to be added.

11 A **False**   normal values are often found in patients with severe
                 abnormalities of extracellular fluid volume.
   B **False**   in chronic hypervolaemia the CVP may not be raised
                 as the bulk of the fluid will lie in the interstitial space
                 rather than in the plasma.
   C **False**   there is often some associated renal failure.
   D **True**   this investigation will reveal extracellular fluid
                 increases prior to the development of pulmonary and
                 sacral oedema. It is particularly useful in the
                 management of chronic hepatic, renal and cardiac
                 problems. In the acutely fluid depleted patient,
                 however, all these factors (A to D) are helpful in
                 assessing fluid requirements.

12 A **False**   this is the definition of oliguria. Anuria is defined as
                 the production of less than 100 ml/day.
   B **False**   in the absence of hypovolaemia immediate fluid
                 restriction should be instituted.
   C **False**   there is almost always overhydration, relative
                 haemodilution and a low serum sodium level.
   D **False**   most patients should have precise fluid therapy based
                 on a policy of replacing only insensible and urinary
                 losses. Cases of refractory renal tubular necrosis may
                 be considered for short term dialysis.

13 A **False**   only insensible losses should be replaced. These will
                 range from 400 to 700 ml/day.
   B **True**   a rising serum potassium is one of the more serious
                 effects of anuria. When it rises above 6 mEq (6mmol)/l
                 exchange resins should be administered orally or
                 rectally and dialysis considered.
   C **False**   metabolic acidosis is almost always present and is
                 due to the accumulation of sulphates and phosphates.
   D **False**   catheterisation should be avoided unless specific
                 surgical indications are present. This will reduce the
                 risk of urinary infection.

14   Acute post-traumatic renal failure
    A   may be due to hypovolaemia and poor tissue perfusion
    B   is particularly associated with crush injuries
    C   may be due to kidney damage following tubular obstruction
    D   should initially be treated by fluid restriction

15   Intravenous parenteral feeding
    A   should deliver at least 2500 calories (10 500J) day to an adult
    B   should deliver at least 10 g of nitrogen
        (i.e. 66 g of protein)/day to an adult
    C   can be effectively achieved with isotonic solutions
    D   is without complications with present day solutions and
        methods of administration

16   Tube feeding of a complete low residue diet
    A   results in constipation
    B   often results in uraemia and dehydration
    C   carries the risk of gastric reflux and pulmonary complications
    D   is ineffective as a long term method of nutrition

14 A **True**   any prolonged decrease in extracellular fluid volume
    B **True**   and tissue perfusion will result in renal dysfunction.
    C **True**   This may also be due to tubular obstruction by blood
                   pigments following crush injuries, mismatched
                   transfusions or burns.
    D **False**   it is desirable to give a provocative test, such as 1 litre
                   of dextrose intravenously in 90 minutes where
                   hypovolaemia is suspected. Similarly, the initial
                   treatment of tubular necrosis should include a fluid
                   load and diuretics. Only when these methods fail
                   should fluids be restricted.

15 A **True**   the ideal solution has not yet been found but the
    B **True**   proteins should be in the form of amino acids and the
                   calorie source as carbohydrate and, to a lesser extent,
                   alcohol. Emulsified fat may also be used.
    C **False**   the tolerable limit for water intake in a sick patient is of
                   the order of 3 litres; thus the solutions used, in order
                   to supply the requisite amount of calories and amino
                   acids must be hypertonic.
    D **False**   thrombophlebitis and septicaemia are frequent
                   complications, diminished to some extent by the use
                   of large veins and the use of a scrupulous sterile
                   technique when setting up the infusion.
                   Hyperosmolar coma is occasionally seen.

16 A **False**   diarrhoea is common with hyperosmolar diets. It
                   should be treated by reducing the rate of
                   administration.
    B **True**   the feeds are often hyperosmolar and excessive fluid
                   losses in the faeces and urine may produce prerenal
                   uraemia and dehydration.
    C **True**   Rapid administration of fluid may be accompanied by
                   regurgitation and aspiration of gastric contents.
    D **False**   with due precautions to avoid the above
                   complications, this is a satisfactory method for long
                   term nutrition.

2 Shock and blood transfusion

17 'Shock' can be most comprehensively defined as
   A a sudden large volume blood loss
   B a diminished effective circulating fluid volume
   C a hypotensive state with peripheral vasoconstriction
   D an unexpected psychological insult

18 In all forms of shock there is
   A an impairment of cellular oxygenation
   B a decreased cardiac output
   C a diminished effective circulating fluid volume
   D a low central venous pressure (CVP)

19 The pulmonary insufficiency, frequently seen in shock, may be caused by
   A an increased pulmonary capillary permeability
   B cardiac failure
   C fluid overload
   D a reduced minute volume

20 Important and urgent measures in the diagnosis and treatment of shock are
   A warming the patient
   B measurement of the central venous pressure
   C noting the response of the central venous pressure to a rapid infusion of 200 to 500 ml of fluid
   D urinary catheterisation

21 The metabolic acidosis of shock can be effectively treated by
   A warming the patient
   B administering sodium bicarbonate
   C artificial ventilation
   D restoring normal tissue perfusion

· 17 A **False**   this definition is incomplete. It does not include shock
due to plasma or water loss, cardiogenic causes or
shock which accompanies generalised septicaemia.
B **True**   this is the most comprehensive definition.
C **False**   early bacteraemic shock is often characterised by
warm extremities.
D **False**   this lay use of the term is irrelevant in the clinical
situation.

18 A **True**   this is present in all forms of shock.
B **False**   the cardiac output is raised in early septicaemic shock.
C **True**   this is a comprehensive definition of the syndrome.
D **False**   in cases of cardiogenic shock the CVP is usually
elevated.

19 A **True**   no single cause of the shock lung has been identified.
B **True**   All these factors together with fat embolism, oxygen
C **True**   toxicity and multiple microemboli in the pulmonary
vessels may play a part. The frequent finding of
pulmonary oedema in the absence of a raised central
venous pressure or a decreased serum albumin,
suggests that increased capillary permeability is the
major cause. In cardiogenic shock and late
hypovolaemia, cardiac failure plays a part. Fluid
overload may occur and produce pulmonary oedema
without right heart failure.
D **False**   the patient is usually hyperventilating and the minute
volume is increased.

20 A **False**   though the skin vessels are usually contracted and the
extremities cold this should be recognised as an effect
rather than the cause of shock. Effective treatment will
restore normal circulation.
B **True**   it is important to ensure that the right atrial filling
C **True**   pressure is sufficient to produce a normal cardiac
D **True**   output. The response of the central venous pressure
to a rapid fluid infusion is often necessary to
distinguish cardiogenic from other forms of shock and
normally the hourly urine volume will drop below 50
ml/hour when inadequate tissue perfusion is present.

21 A **False**   the basic cause of the acidosis is poor tissue perfusion
B **True**   and unless this is corrected there can be no
C **False**   permanent improvement. Bicarbonate is only
D **True**   necessary in cases of severe acidosis when a pH of
below 7.1 may lead to serious cardiac arrhythmias.

22   In hypovolaemic shock
   A   the central venous pressure is low
   B   the difference in arteriovenous oxygen tension is unaffected
   C   the extremities are pale, cold and sweating
   D   urine output is unaffected

23   Hypovolaemic shock may result from
   A   a 25 per cent third degree burn
   B   generalised peritonitis
   C   massive pulmonary embolism
   D   intestinal obstruction

24   Appropriate *immediate* intravenous infusions in all cases of non-cardiogenic shock are
   A   whole blood
   B   ringer's lactate
   C   normal saline
   D   low molecular weight dextran

25   Oliguria occurring in a shocked patient after the central venous pressure and blood pressure have been corrected to normal may require
   A   frusemide 40 mg intravenously
   B   mannitol 20 g in 200 ml 5 per cent dextrose
   C   an increased fluid intake
   D   potassium supplements

22 A **True**   this is due to the low circulating fluid volume.
   B **False**   the associated decreased cardiac output leads to an increased arteriovenous difference in oxygen tension.
   C **True**   this is due to reflex sympathetic stimulae.
   D **False**   the hourly urine volume falls because of decreased renal perfusion. Treatment should aim to maintain urine outflow at about 50 ml/hr.

23 A **True**   this is due to excessive sequestration of fluid in the burned area and to serum losses.
   B **True**   this is due to fluid sequestration in the inflamed peritoneum and adynamic bowel.
   C **False**   there is no change in the extracellular volume in this condition although cardiogenic shock frequently follows the reduced cardiac output.
   D **True**   hypovolaemia results from excessive fluid loss due to fluid sequestration in the distended bowel.

24 A **False**   this should be restricted to cases of blood loss.
   B **True**   both of these isotonic fluids satisfactorily expand the
   C **True**   plasma volume. The serum electrolytes should be estimated as soon as possible to assess the long term requirements. The haematocrit should be checked to assess the need for blood.
   D **True**   though this fluid has few advantages over Ringer's lactate or saline and can produce spontaneous bleeding and crossmatching problems.

25 A **True**   Both these diuretics can be used. If there is no diuresis
   B **True**   after 30 minutes, frusemide may then be given again in a dose of up to 600 mg. If there is still no effect serious renal damage should be suspected and a regime of fluid restriction instituted.
   C **False**   this may result in fluid overload.
   D **False**   serum potassium levels rise in renal failure and may be lethal.

**26   The following vasoactive drugs may be used intravenously with
        benefit in the shocked patient**
    A adrenaline
    B noradrenaline
    C isoprenaline
    D phenoxybenzamine

27   Septic shock
    A is only caused by gram-negative organisms
    B carries a favourable prognosis
    C produces a cellular defect that inhibits oxygen utilisation
    D is particularly associated with infective complications of the
        gastrointestinal and genito-urinary systems

28   Septic shock is particularly associated with
    A thoracic surgical patients
    B hypovolaemia
    C indwelling urinary or intravenous catheters
    D gram-negative bacteraemia

29   Early septic shock is commonly associated with
    A a high central venous pressure
    B a high cardiac output
    C a low blood pressure
    D cold sweaty extremities

**30   The presence of spontaneous haemorrhage in septic shock
        suggests**
    A hypovolaemia
    B liver failure
    C excessive fibrinolysis
    D disseminated intravascular coagulation (DIC)

26 A **False** — both these drugs increase peripheral resistance and
   B **False** — decrease cardiac output. Their use in shock is detrimental. Intracardiac adrenaline may be used in the treatment of ventricular asystole.
   C **True** — in some forms of cardiogenic shock (where bradycardia is present) and in advanced hypovolaemic shock with associated heart failure this drug may be helpful.
   D **True** — this vasodilator may increase cardiac output. It should only be given to patients who are not hypovolaemic and whose CVP is being monitored.

27 A **False** — although the commonest organisms are gram-negative, gram-positive organisms and fungi may also cause septic shock.
   B **False** — the mortality usually exceeds 30 per cent.
   C **True** — this may precede the haemodynamic changes.
   D **True** — this incidence is further increased by instrumental or surgical manipulation of the infected region.

28 A **False** — both medical and surgical patients are at risk,
   B **True** — particularly those with hypovolaemia, septic foci and
   C **True** — indwelling intravenous cannulae or urinary catheters.
   D **True** — 30 per cent of patients with a gram-negative bacteraemia develop septic shock and this is commoner in patients with widespread neoplasia and in patients over the age of 50.

29 A **True** — hyperdynamic or 'warm' shock is a frequent early
   B **True** — pattern in septic shock. This is associated with
   C **True** — hyperventilation and a low blood pressure the
   D **False** — extremities are warm and dry due to vasodilatation and a higher than normal cardiac output.

30 A **False** — not associated
   B **False** — not associated
   C **True** — endotoxin may accelerate the clotting process to
   D **True** — produce DIC which in its turn can produce spontaneous haemorrhages, pulmonary oedema and pancreatitis. Excessive fibrinolysis may be associated with DIC, but may occur independently. Treatment of DIC may require fresh blood transfusions and possibly heparinisation.

31 **Septic shock is associated with a hypodynamic cardiovascular state**
   A if preceded by existing hypovolaemia
   B in generalised peritonitis
   C when there is a gram-positive bacteraemia
   D in elderly patients

32 **The diminished oxygen consumption in patients with septic shock is due to**
   A failure of oxygen transport in the lungs
   B diminished blood flow in the periphery
   C arteriovenous shunting in the periphery
   D diminished oxygen utilisation by the cells

33 **The mortality from septic shock can be effectively reduced by**
   A surgical drainage of abscesses
   B the administration of appropriate antibiotics
   C the restoration of a normal cardiovascular state
   D positive pressure respiration via a tracheostomy

34 **In cardiogenic shock**
   A the central venous pressure is low
   B the difference in the arteriovenous oxygen tension is increased
   C the haematocrit is raised
   D the blood pressure is unaffected

35 **Prospective blood donors**
   A should be asked about previous attacks of jaundice
   B should have serological tests for syphilis
   C may transmit glandular fever to a recipient
   D may transmit malaria to a recipient

31 A **True**   in all cases where sepsis complicates a process
    B **True**   producing a loss of extracellular fluid volume such as
                      peritonitis, gangrenous bowel and intestinal
                      obstruction, the hypodynamic pattern of shock is seen
                      with a low central venous pressure, low cardiac
                      output and cold sweaty extremities.
    C **False**   this form of septic shock characteristically produces a
                      hyperdynamic state.
    D **True**   these patients are particularly prone to septic shock.

32 A **True**   the pulmonary oedema associated with septic shock
                      impairs oxygen uptake.
    B **False**   even in hyperdynamic states, where peripheral blood
                      flow is increased, there is a deficient oxygen uptake
                      due to impaired cellular functions.
    C **False**   xenon clearance studies have not shown any
                      peripheral arteriovenous shunting in these patients.
    D **True**   vital cell functions are impaired with a resultant
                      inability to utilise oxygen.

33 A **True**   patients have a better prognosis after drainage.
    B **True**   the mortality rate is halved when effective antibiotics
                      are used.
    C **True**   this may require blood or saline infusions and
                      possibly the administration of isoprenaline and
                      digitalis.
    D **True**   mechanical ventilation should not be restricted to
                      those patients with specific respiratory indications.

34 A **False**   there is usually an increased central venous pressure.
    B **True**   this is due to inadequate tissue perfusion.
    C **False**   the haematocrit is unchanged whereas in
                      hypovolaemic shock not due to blood loss it is raised.
    D **False**   the inadequate cardiac output always produces a fall
                      in blood pressure.

35 A **True**   Donors who have had serum or infective hepatitis
                      may remain infective for up to 3 years.
    B **True**   spirochaetes are transmissible (they will survive for 4
                      days in stored blood). Gonorrhoea is not
                      transmissible.
    C **True**   this infection is transmissible.
    D **True**   in some countries malarial donors are not accepted
                      although the serum alone may be used without risk of
                      transmission.

36   A blood transfusion reaction
    A may be due to incompatibility of the recipient serum and donor cells
    B is manifest by thrombophlebitis of the infusion site
    C occurs within the first 30 minutes of transfusion
    D may produce renal damage

37   Pyrexial reactions to blood transfusions
    A have increased since the introduction of sterile disposable infusion sets
    B may be caused by allergic reactions
    C may be caused by contaminated blood
    D may be a response to a large transfusion of cooled blood

38   Massive blood transfusions may be complicated by
    A hyperkalaemia
    B hypercalcaemia
    C hepatic coma
    D leucopenia

36 A **True**   mismatching produces agglutination of the donor cells.
    B **False**   the signs include fever, chills, breathlessness and pain in the flanks and chest. These may be followed by hypotension, haemorrhagic phenomena and haemoglobinuria.
    C **True**   this period should be closely observed when a blood transfusion is commenced.
    D **true**   this is the result of haemoglobinuria, hypotension and acidosis. It should be treated by immediately stopping the transfusion, invoking a diuresis and restoring the patient's blood pressure.

37 A **False**   pyrogen reactions have decreased since the introduction of disposable infusion sets.
    B **True**   this is due to allergens in the donor blood
    C **True**   gram-negative endotoxins are the commonest cause and bacteria may multiply in warm blood. Blood should therefore be stored at 4°C until it is required.
    D **False**   this produces a fall in body temperature.

38 A **True**   in 3-week-old blood the plasma potassium rises to 30 to 40 mEq (30 to 40 mmol)/litre.
    B **False**   hypocalcaemia may occur and this is accentuated if citrate is used as the anticoagulant. It should be treated by the administration of calcium chloride.
    C **True**   this may occur in cirrhotic patients, possibly due to a high ammonia concentration.
    D **False**   there is no change in the white cell count.

3 Burns

39 **When determining the depth of a burn**
   A a knowledge of the type of injury is important
   B the presence of blisters is of no clinical significance
   C impairment of sensibility of the burned area should be tested
   D the presence of severe pain denotes a full thickness skin loss

40 **Estimation of the area of a burn**
   A is of very little clinical significance
   B provides important prognostic information
   C is an important factor in the estimation of the fluid required
   D can be based on a formula which states that the adult trunk is
       36 per cent of the whole body surface area

41 **Patients with major burns**
   A are in a negative nitrogen balance
   B have normal calorie requirements
   C do not generally become anaemic
   D are resistant to septicaemia

42 **The catabolic response to trauma and infection is characterised by**
   A an increase in lean body mass
   B a positive nitrogen balance
   C gluconeogenesis
   D a falling haemoglobin level

39 A **True**   contact with hot liquids usually causes partial
                   thickness loss, whereas flames commonly give rise to
                   full thickness losses.
   B **False**   blisters do not occur in full thickness loss.
   C **True**   full thickness burns have a reduced pain sensibility.
   D **False**   nerve endings in the area of a full thickness burn are
                   usually destroyed.

40 A **False**   the form of therapy and the fluid requirements of the
                   patient are determined by the area of the burn.
   B **True**   the prognosis after a burn injury is related to the
                   extent of the burn.
   C **True**   this is an important guide, although no formula for
                   fluid therapy in burns can be precise. It is also
                   important to carefully monitor indices of tissue
                   perfusion and cardiovascular status, such as hourly
                   urine volume and central venous pressure
                   measurements.
   D **True**   the 'Rule of Nines' wherein the head and upper limbs
                   each measure 9 per cent and the lower limbs 18 per
                   cent each is widely used as a rough guide in
                   estimating the area of a burn.

41 A **True**   even if the greatly increased needs of 150 to 200 g
                   protein/day are met the negative nitrogen balance will
                   persist until the wound is healed.
   B **False**   calorie requirements may be at least twice normal due
                   to increased energy losses such as through increased
                   evaporative water loss and fever. Parenteral nutrition
                   is thus frequently necessary.
   C **False**   there is blood destruction and sequestration in the
                   early days of a burn. These factors together with
                   infection and septicaemia give rise to anaemia.
   D **False**   they have an increased subsceptibility to infection and
                   have many more potential sources of infection than a
                   healthy patient.

42 A **False**   a breakdown of tissue protein provides substrates for
                   gluconeogenesis.
   B **False**   there is thus a loss of most body tissue proteins, this
                   being reflected.
   C **True**   by a decrease of the lean body mass and a negative
                   nitrogen balance.
   D **False**   haemoglobin synthesis is usually unaffected in the
                   catabolic phase.

43   The catabolic response to trauma
  A   is related to the severity of the trauma
  B   is accompanied by increased urinary losses of potassium and nitrogen
  C   can be prevented by parenteral nutrition
  D   does not occur in the adrenalectomised patient

44   Scalds
  A   are more frequent in children
  B   commonly cause full thickness skin loss
  C   should be skin grafted within 48 hours of the injury
  D   need routine antibiotic treatment

45   The dressing of a small burn should be
  A   occlusive
  B   non-absorbtive
  C   non-compressive
  D   changed daily as a routine

46   A partial thickness burn
  A   may heal without grafting
  B   may deteriorate into full thickness skin loss
  C   rarely causes severe physiological derangement of the patient
  D   heals within 7 days in the absence of infection

43 A **True**   whereas a patient with a fractured femur will lose approximately 11 g of nitrogen (70 g of protein)/day, a major burn may lose 40 g of nitrogen/day.

  B **True**   following protein catabolism and gluconeogenesis.

  C **False** parenterally administered amino acids when suitably admixed with a source of calories minimise but do not abolish the catabolic response.

  D **False** there is no known dependance on the endocrine system.

44 A **True**   this is especially so in children under 3 years of age.

  B **False** hot or boiling water usually produces partial skin loss.

  C **False** local cleansing and the application of a non-adherent

  D **False** sterile dressing are all that is usually required. Healing generally takes place uneventfully without the need for grafting or antibiotic therapy.

45 A **True**   the aim of the dressing is to prevent bacterial invasion

  B **False** and to provide firm compression and support. If these

  C **False** criteria are met, it need only be changed every 4 or 5

  D **False** days. The infected burn will require dressing daily or more frequently.

46 A **True**   epithelial regeneration will spread from the epithelial remnants in the hair follicles and deeper layers of the epidermis.

  B **True**   infection may convert it into a full thickness skin loss by destroying the remaining dermal elements.

  C **false** in a deep partial thickness burn there is a considerable inflammatory response even though some epidermal elements may have escaped injury. If the burn is of more than 15 to 20 per cent of the body surface, hypovolaemia may develop.

  D **False** the deeper partial thickness burns may require 3 or 4 weeks before epithelial regeneration is complete.

47 Fluid losses in a major burn
  A are maximal between 12 and 24 hours after the injury
  B are related to the age of the patient
  C are related to the weight of the patient
  D are related to the area burnt

48 The increased fluid requirements of a patient with a full thickness burn are due to
  A increased evaporative water loss
  B sequestration of fluid in the injured tissues
  C serum exuding from the burned area
  D destruction of blood in the skin vessels

49 48 hours after a major burn and with satisfactory fluid therapy a patient
  A has very few abnormal fluid losses
  B may need a blood transfusion
  C is often hypernatraemic
  D usually needs skin grafting

47 A **False**   are maximal in the first 8 hours after burning.
    B **False**   there is no known relationship to age but there is a
    C **True**   direct relationship to body weight, the area burnt and
    D **True**   the depth of the burn. Many guides to fluid therapy in
                   the burned patient take account of these factors, e.g:
                   First 24 hours:
                     (i) electrolyte solution 1.5 ml/kg/per cent body
                        surface burn
                     (ii) colloid solution 0.5 ml/kg/per cent body surface
                        burn.
                   Plus metabolic requirements (approximately 2000
                   ml in an adult). Half the above fluid is given
                   intravenously in the first 8 hours and one-quarter in
                   each of the successive 8 hours.

48 A **True**   evaporative water loss from a full thickness burn is
    B **True**   more than 10 times that of intact skin. Two and a half
    C **True**   litres of water may be lost per day from a 40 per cent
                  burn. There is a local (and to a lesser extent, a general)
                  increase in capillary permeability so that protein-rich
                  fluid gains the interstitial space from the blood. Large
                  amounts of fluid are sequestrated in the inflammation
                  which surrounds the burn injury. Relatively little
                  serum is lost from a full thickness burn.
    D **False** although there is some destruction of red cells and a
                  diminution in the red cell mass this is not an important
                  factor in accounting for the increased fluid
                  requirements.

49 A **False** insensible evaporative water loss is still excessive —
                  up to 3 litres/day in the adult with extensive burns.
    B **True**   destruction of red cells, trapping of blood in
                  thrombosed capillaries and increased phagocytosis of
                  red cells may produce anaemia at this time.
    C **True**   this is mainly due to increased insensible losses of
                  water.
    D **False** surgical debridement of a major burn at this time is
                  very traumatic and is rarely indicated. Skin grafting is
                  sometimes undertaken after 7 days but there is a need
                  for great care in limiting the blood loss.

50   Major burns are sometimes complicated by
    A acute gastric and duodenal ulcers
    B paralytic ileus
    C cerebral oedema
    D mesenteric thrombosis

51   In a burned patient, associated pulmonary injury
    A should be suspected in head and neck burns
    B should be suspected when the nasal hairs are burnt
    C does not appear clinically in the first 24 hours
    D may be avoided by the prophylactic use of antibiotics

52   Secondary infection of burns
    A is less common in partial than in full thickness skin loss
    B is relatively more common in burns of more than 20 per cent body area
    C is avoided by leaving the burn eschar intact
    D is avoided by the immediate application of a sterile occlusive dressing

53   The early management of a burn wound may include
    A early excision
    B occlusive dressings
    C exposure treatment
    D dressings with local antibiotics

50 A **True**   the ulcers are known as Curling's ulcers. They are
                     frequently multiple in the stomach and most common
                     in extensive burns.
    B **True**   this often lasts 48 to 72 hours.
    C **True**   this is maximal 48 to 72 hours after the injury when
                     the risk of hyponatraemia due to over-transfusion
                     with intravenous fluids is greatest.
    D **False**   there is no recognised relationship.

51 A **True**   the additional sign of pharyngeal inflammation may
    B **True**   be present and should be looked for.
    C **False**   the effects of burn injury to the lungs are often
                     immediate.
    D **False**   antibiotics do not prevent the injury but may prevent
                     secondary infection.

52 A **True**   the protective function of the skin against invasive
    B **False**   infection by environmental organisms is lost when a
                     full thickness burn is present. To a large extent this
                     protective function is retained in a partial thickness
                     burn. Small burns are as readily infected as large
                     burns.
    C **False**   the dry dead burn eschar is permeable and is an entry
                     site for invasive infection.
    D **False**   viable bacteria may remain in the follicles deep to the
                     burned surface and subsequently multiply to infect
                     the area.

53 A **True**   all these treatments are acceptable depending on the
    B **True**   type of burn minor partial thickness burns may
    C **True**   warrant outpatient management with occlusive
    D **True**   dressings and small full thickness burns early
                     excision. In major burns fluid therapy has priority and
                     the burn is treated as the circumstances dictate.

54   Skin grafting of a burn wound
  A should usually be with full thickness skin grafts
  B is more likely to be successful if undertaken in the first week after injury
  C will be unsuccessful unless the wound surface is sterile
  D minimises scar contracture

55   The prognosis of a burned patient is
  A related to the patient's age
  B related to the area burnt
  C generally better below the age of 10 years
  D very poor in the patient with burns of over 40 per cent surface area

54 A **False**   with the exception of very small burns of the eyelids
                     or the delayed treatment of contractures (when full
                     thickness pedicle grafts may be used), split thickness
                     skin grafts are used.
    B **False**   grafting is less successful before granulation tissue is
                     present. However homo- or hetero-graft skin may be
                     used as a very effective burn dressing in the early
                     stages of repair.
    C **False**   although beta-haemolytic streptococci are inimical to
                     skin grafts, moderate infections of the wound with
                     other organisms are not a contra-indication to skin
                     grafting.
    D **True**   for this reason burns around joints should receive
                     early attention.

55 A **True**   after middle age the prognosis worsens with
                     advancing years.
    B **True**   there is a direct relationship; the larger the burn the
                     worse the prognosis.
    C **False**   young children have a higher mortality rate than
                     adults in burns of equivalent size.
    D **False**   40 per cent survival rates have been recorded in series
                     of patients with 60 per cent burns and occasional
                     survivors are reported in patients with more than 70
                     per cent burns.

4 Wound Healing, Surgical Infection and Postoperative Complications

56 A clean incised skin wound
   A undergoes an inflammatory phase during the processes of repair
   B commences epithelialization after 7 to 10 days
   C regains the full strength of normal skin within 10 days
   D regains its strength as the result of fibroblast activity

57 Wound healing
   A is impaired in anaemic patients
   B is impaired by haematoma formation
   C is impaired by hypoproteinaemia
   D is stimulated by steroids

58 The principles of wound care include
   A early skin cover
   B removal of foreign material
   C routine administration of antibiotics
   D close apposition of uninfected wounded tissues

59 Heavily contaminated and dirty wounds
   A require surgical toilet and delayed closure
   B require the administration of systemic antibiotics
   C can usually be treated by wound toilet and primary closure
   D should be totally excised

56 A **True**   polymorphs and monocytes accumulate and engulf
                     cell debris and all foreign material during the initial
                     phase of repair.
    B **False**   a clean incised wound whose edges are opposed is
                     re-epithelialized within 2 days.
    C **False**   healed skin wounds are never as strong as
                     unwounded skin. After 8 weeks it has reached 80 per
                     cent of its original strength.
    D **True**   These cells synthesise collagen.

57 A **False**   no studies have confirmed this widely held view.
    B **True**   any foreign material, fluid or haematoma prolongs the
                     inflammatory phase and inhibits fibroblast invasion.
    C **True**   an albumin concentration below 2.5 g/100 ml
                     significantly impairs wound healing.
    D **False**   steroids decrease the rate of epithelialization and
                     inhibit fibroblast proliferation. They thus have an
                     inhibitory effect on wound healing.

58 A **True**   the principles of meticulous debridement and careful
    B **True**   tissue apposition should be adhered to whether the
    C **False**   wound is from a sterile surgical knife or is the untidy
    D **True**   contaminated wound of a road traffic accident. Skin
                     grafts should cover skin defects as soon as possible.
                     When wound toilet is not possible within 12 to 18
                     hours it is usually best to delay closure of the wound
                     because by this time active bacterial multiplication
                     has occurred. Antibiotics should only be used when
                     infection is likely to have occurred.

59 A **True**   meticulous removal of dead and foreign material
    B **True**   coupled with the administration of a suitable broad
    C **False**   spectrum antibiotic and gentle packing with gauze
                     prior to delayed closure 4 or 5 days later is the most
                     effective form of treatment.
    D **False**   the remaining wound would be scarcely less
                     contaminated and such radical therapy is usually only
                     necessary in spreading infections such as gas
                     gangrene.

60 Surgical drainage of abscesses
A should be via a small incision with minimal disturbance of the adjacent tissues
B should be dependent wherever possible
C has been outmoded by antibiotic therapy
D should be undertaken before the signs of fluctuation appear

61 In localised surgical infections
A an elevated leucocyte count is usually present
B fever and tenderness are usually present
C the presence of glycosuria usually indicates matastatic pancreatic abscesses
D pus is frequently absent

62 Staphylococcal infections
A do not cause cellulitis
B do not produce septicaemia
C do not produce fever
D produce yellow odourless pus

63 Streptococcal infections
A are characterised by abscess formation
B rarely produce lymphadenitis
C frequently produce bacteraemia
D can produce a gangrenous skin infection

64 Tetanus prophylaxis in a patient with a badly contaminated wound
A depends, even in an actively immunised patient, on meticulous immediate debridement of the wound
B should include the administration of tetanus toxoid
C is more safely achieved with equine rather than human antitoxin
D is unnecessary in patients who have been recently actively immunised

60 A **False**   bold incisions, with the breaking down of all loculi and
the removal of slough should be undertaken.
    B **True**   gravity will help drainage.
    C **False**   antibiotics are of little value in the treatment of an
abscess but when cellulitis surrounds the abscess,
they should be used as an adjunct to surgery.
    D **False**   at this point the infection may be at the cellulitic stage
and not localised. It is then justifiable to administer
antibiotics and carefully observe the response.
(Fluctuation is, of course, only elicited in palpable
abscesses.)

61 A **True**   in an infection attenuated by prolonged and partially
    B **True**   effective antibiotic therapy these common signs are
frequently absent.
    C **False**   diabetes and infection do however frequently co-exist
and make the treatment of each more difficult.
    D **False**   it is a characteristic of all localised infections that pus
(necrotic cellular debris, macrophages and bacteria) is
found surrounded by granulation tissue and fibrosis
(the abscess wall).

62 A **False**   staphylococcal cellulitis does occur.
    B **False**   septicaemia does occur and may be accompanied by
septic shock and matastatic abscess formation.
    C **False**   pyrexia is present in all but the smallest skin eruptions.
    D **True**   this characterises a staphylococcal abscess.

63 A **False**   they are characteristically invasive and produce
cellulitis.
    B **False**   lymphangitis and lymphadenitis are common.
    C **True**   this should be suspected when pyrexia, rigor or
toxaemia develops.
    D **True**   streptococcal gangrene, due to anaerobic organisms,
is characterised by oedema and haemorrhagic skin
bullae. It may be confused with a clostridial cellulitis.

64 A **True**   this is *essential* and cannot be over-emphasised.
    B **True**   the previously unimmunised patient should also
receive antitetanus toxin; the actively immunised
patient requires a booster dose of toxoid.
    C **False**   the antibody titre remains higher for a longer period
with the human antitoxin. The equine variety is
complicated by allergic reactions and cross-sensitivity
in about half the patients.
    D **False**   see B—prophylaxis should *always* include wound
care.

65   Tetanus
   A may have an incubation period of over 20 days
   B can be prevented by the immediate administration of tetanus
      toxoid
   C is more common after scalp lacerations than wounds of the
      extremities
   D is usually associated with stupor or coma

66   The treatment of established tetanus
   A should include wound excision
   B has been improved by the use of mechanical ventilation
   C requires adequate and prolonged antibiotic therapy
   D should include treatment with human antitetanus antitoxin

67   Clostridial myositis
   A is otherwise known as gas gangrene
   B has a 2 to 3 week incubation period
   C may produce jaundice
   D may rapidly produce anaemia

68   In clostridial infections
   A a spreading cellulitis may be present
   B gram-positive cocci can be isolated from the discharge
   C surgical treatment has a minor part to play
   D gas production is often absent

65 A **True**   this may vary from 3 to 24 days.
   B **False** active immunisation will not confer protection for 2 to 3 weeks after the injection of the toxoid. Wounds which are contaminated with foreign bodies or necrotic tissue are particularly at risk. Prophylaxis should include adequate wound toilet and passive immunisation of the previously unimmunised patient. Patients who have had a full course of active immunisation with toxoid require a booster dose.
   C **False** injuries of the extremities are more frequently complicated by tetanus. The rich blood supply of the scalp confers some protection.
   D **False** the patient's conscious level is rarely depressed.

66 A **True**   this will prevent the release of further exotoxins.
   B **True**   the spasms and clonic contractions that characterise the severe infection are painful, distressing and may interfere with respiration. Thus, these cases may need treatment with muscle relaxants, sedatives and mechanical ventilation.
   C **False** although antibiotics may be required for the initial treatment of the causative wound, they are ineffective in the treatment of established tetanus.
   D **True**   the human, rather than the equine, antitoxin allows successive doses of antitoxin to be given sub-cutaneously and systemically. It has improved the results of treatment.

67 A **True**   it is caused most frequently by *C.welchii* and *C.septicum*.
   B **False** this is a very rapidly progressive infection generally associated with a poor blood supply and delayed surgical care to contaminated wounds.
   C **True**   the many clostridial exotoxins giving rise to severe
   D **True**   systemic effects include potent haemolysins.

68 A **True**   *Clostridium welchii* may cause this serious condition. It is characterised by a rapidly spreading crepitant cellulitis.
   B **False** Clostridia are gram-positive rod shaped bacilli.
   C **False** early desloughing, wound toilet and surgical de-compression by incision and fasciotomy are essential. Antibiotics are an adjunct to surgery.
   D **True**   *Clostridium tetani* does not generally produce gas and gas production in *Clostridium welchii* cellulitis and myositis may be absent. Streptococcal cellulitis and mixed infections sometimes produce gas in the tissues.

69   Actinomycosis is characterised by
   A   chronic abscesses of the cervico-facial region
   B   a granulomatous abscess wall
   C   red coloured pus
   D   its resistance to antibiotics

70   A subphrenic abscess
   A   is usually accompanied by considerable systemic effects
   B   is associated with local rib tenderness
   C   rarely produces abnormal signs in the chest
   D   may be diagnosed by a barium meal examination

71   A pelvic abscess
   A   lies extraperitoneally
   B   may be a complication of abdominal surgery
   C   often presents with diarrhoea
   D   should be treated with antibiotics alone

69 A **True**   other common sites are the chest wall and the caecum.
    B **True**   the fibrotic abscess wall contains many granulomata
    C **False**   and tangled masses of branching filaments ('Sulphur'
                     granules) which give a characteristic yellow colour to
                     the pus.
    D **False**   the infection can be effectively treated by a 3 to 4 week
                     course of penicillin or tetracycline.

70 A **False**   the signs and symptoms of this condition are
    B **True**   frequently minimal, with only a mild pyrexia and a
    C **False**   leucocytosis being present. Occasionally there
                     is tenderness between the overlying ribs, a
                     sympathetic pleural effusion in the adjacent pleural
                     cavity, shoulder tip pain and hiccoughs.
    D **True**   a left sided subphrenic abscess may be noted on
                     barium meal by indentation of the fundus of the
                     stomach. The most commonly employed radiological
                     technique is to observe diaphragmatic movement
                     under fluoroscopy. This is diminished on the affected
                     side.

71 A **False**   this abscess lies in the lowest cul-de-sac of
                     peritoneum, the recto-vesical or recto-uterine pouch.
    B **True**   it may also result from an infected neighbouring
                     viscus, e.g. appendix or from generalised peritonitis.
    C **True**   watery diarrhoea frequently results from associated
                     rectal inflammation. The systemic effects of an
                     abscess are also present.
    D **False**   antibiotics are useful when the pelvic infection is at
                     the cellulitic stage and as an adjunct to surgery. They
                     cannot alone treat an established abscess and surgical
                     drainage is required.

72   Paralytic ileus
A   is associated with electrolyte imbalance
B   may be associated with mechanical intestinal obstruction
C   requires treatment with nasogastric suction and intravenous fluids
D   is associated with retroperitoneal haematoma

73   Acute postoperative gastric dilatation
A   may cause postoperative vascular collapse
B   can be prevented by regular nasogastric aspiration
C   characteristically occurs on the first postoperative day
D   is a relatively common problem after surgery on the gastrointestinal tract

74   The appearance of jaundice in the postoperative period
A   may indicate an intraperitoneal haemorrhage
B   is usually due to the toxic effects of anaesthetic agents
C   may be due to septicaemia
D   may indicate chronic liver disease

75   A distal small bowel fistula
A   loses intestinal fluid rich in potassium and sodium
B   may give rise to a metabolic acidosis
C   rapidly results in dehydration
D   may be managed conservatively by the abandonment of oral feeding

72 A **True**   there are abnormal fluid and electrolyte losses in a
   B **True**   patient with paralytic ileus. Hypokalaemia particularly
   C **True**   contributes to further inhibition of intestinal motility
                 by interfering with the normal ionic movements
                 during smooth muscle contraction. Prolonged
                 intestinal distension such as is associated with
                 mechanical intestinal obstruction may also inhibit
                 intestinal motility. Decompression of the distended
                 bowel by nasogastric suction and replacement of the
                 abnormal fluid losses form the basis of treatment after
                 mechanical causes of the obstruction have been ruled
                 out.
   D **True**   retroperitoneal haemorrhage, severe trauma,
                 particularly to the vertebral column, and ureteric
                 distension all inhibit intestinal motility.

73 A **True**   gastric distention (with up to 5 or 6 litres of fluid) is
                 associated with hypovolaemia.
   B **True**   this is frequently undertaken for the first 2 to 3
                 postoperative days until flatus is passed and bowel
                 sounds return to normal.
   C **False**   it usually occurs 2 or 3 days after abdominal
                 operations.
   D **False**   the routine use of postoperative nasogastric suction
                 has almost abolished its incidence after abdominal
                 surgery. It still occurs in severe injuries and burns
                 where nasogastric suction is less commonly used.

74 A **True**   the blood is haemolysed producing a transient mild
                 haemolytic jaundice.
   B **False**   certain anaesthetic agents (such as chloroform and
                 possibly halothane) have a hepatotoxic effect, but the
                 incidence is very low.
   C **True**   severe sepsis may give rise to jaundice, probably by
                 haemolysis.
   D **True**   hypotension and hypoxia during the operative period
                 may precipitate jaundice in a patient with chronic liver
                 disease.

75 A **True**   the concentration of sodium in the fistulous fluid is
                 comparable to plasma and that of potassium often
                 higher.
   B **True**   this is due to the alkaline nature of the fistulous losses.
   C **True**   water losses may be as much as 4 or 5 litres per day.
   D **True**   provided there is no distal obstruction, parenteral
                 nutrition and the cessation of oral feeding may result
                 in a decrease of the fistulous losses and eventual
                 closure.

76   A pancreatic fistula
  A   loses fluids with high potassium and lower sodium levels than plasma
  B   may give rise to a metabolic acidosis
  C   requires long term treatment with intravenous normal saline
  D   will usually close if oral feeding is temporarily suspended

77   Bed sores
  A   can be prevented by sheepskin blankets
  B   can be prevented by changing the patient's position four times each 24 hours.
  C   are the consequence of local infection
  D   only occur over the sacrum

61% on 18/3

76 A **False**   the sodium and potassium levels in pancreatic fluid
                      are similar to those of plasma.
    B **True**   there are high bicarbonate losses.
    C **False**   because of B the patient must be sustained on sodium
                      lactate or bicarbonate solution.
    D **False**   the high concentration of enzymes renders skin
                      excoriation a major problem and abandonment of oral
                      feeding will only slightly diminish the volume of
                      fistula losses. It thus has little effect on the healing of
                      the fistula.

77 A **False**   bed sores are due to local ischaemia. This may occur
    B **False**   over any bony prominences, the back of the head, the
    C **False**   heels and the greater trochanter of the femur as well
    D **False**   as the sacrum. They are often the consequence of
                      inadequate nursing (and medical) care and
                      observation. They are best prevented by changing the
                      patient's position every 2 hours. Sheepskin and foam
                      underlays add support to the nursing endeavours.

5 Skin and breast

78 Maglignant melanomata
- A occur more commonly in the black races
- B occur with equal frequency in all ages
- C frequently arise from pre-existing benign naevi
- D occur more frequently in tropical regions

79 A malignant melanoma
- A frequently arises from hair-bearing naevi
- B frequently arises from junctional naevi
- C has a worse prognosis when it arises on the leg
- D should be suspected in any pigmented lesion which bleeds spontaneously

80 The treatment of a malignant melanoma should include
- A a preliminary incision biopsy
- B wide excision of the tumour
- C 'en bloc' removal of adjacent involved lymph nodes
- D immediate excision of any enlarging lymph node in the postoperative period

78 A **False**   these are rare in the black races where they are usually found only in the depigmented skin of the feet and hands.

B **False**   they usually present between the ages of 30 and 60. They are very rare in the prepubertal child.

C **True**   approximately half the patients give a history of change in a preexisting stable pigmented lesion.

D **True**   the incidence in the white races is related quite closely to the amount of solar radiation received. The highest incidence is in white Australians.

79 A **False**   these naevi contain dermal elements and have a very low malignant potential.

B **True**   these flat, usually darkly pigmented lesions are those most likely to undergo malignant change.

C **False**   lower limb melanomata have the best prognosis. Head, neck and trunk melanomata have the worst. Late recognition is thought to be a factor in explaining the poor survival of the latter group.

D **True**   this is a warning sign, together with itching, ulceration, progressive growth and increased pigmentation.

80 A **False**   dissemination by blood and lymphatic systems frequently follows this procedure.

B **True**   the extent of the excision is related to the size and site of the primary, but many authorities state that a 5 cm margin of normal tissue is the minimum to be excised.

C **True**   but the policy regarding 'prophylactic' lymph node removal when they are remote from the tumour and possibly uninvolved is less certain and much controversy exists.

D **True**   examinations should be carried out every 1 to 3 months for at least the first 2 years. Enlargement of regional nodes is then noted early and is an indication for immediate excision of those nodes. In this way systemic spread can be avoided in some patients.

81   **Squamous cancer of the lip**
     A   is most common in early adult life
     B   is more common in fair skinned subjects
     C   metastasises readily by the blood stream
     D   is preferably treated by radiotherapy once lymph node
         deposits are present

82   **Basal cell carcinomas**
     A   usually metastasise to regional lymph nodes
     B   are less common than squamous cell carcinomas
     C   are characterised histologically by epithelial pearls
     D   are particularly common in oriental races

83   **Capillary angiomas of childhood (strawberry naevi)**
     A   arise in the dermis
     B   are premalignant
     C   are most satisfactorily treated with superficial radiotherapy
     D   should be surgically excised

84   **Fibroadenomata of the breast**
     A   are commonest in early adult life
     B   are indiscrete and difficult to distinguish
     C   are usually painless
     D   resolve without treatment

81 A **False**   there is an increasing incidence with age. It is
   B **True**   particularly common in people exposed to large
                  amounts of sunlight particularly if their skin has little
                  natural pigmentation. It is very rare in the black races.
   C **False**   the most common mode of spread is by direct
                  extension to neighbouring tissues. Lymphatic spread
                  does occur, particularly in poorly differentiated
                  lesions, but spread via the blood stream is
                  uncommon.
   D **False**   surgical excision is recommended with block
                  dissection of the neck if there is evidence of lymph
                  node metastasis. Radiotherapy on its own is indicated
                  for small well-differentiated lesions, when the
                  possibility of metastasis is unlikely, or as palliative
                  treatment in the late stages of the disease.

82 A **False**   while this is so in squamous cell carcinomata,
                  metastases are very rare in basal cell lesions.
   B **False**   they are approximately three times more common.
   C **False**   these are characteristic of squamous cell carcinomas.
                  The classical appearance in basal cell lesions is of
                  darkly staining solid masses of cells arising from the
                  basal layer of epidermis.
   D **False**   such lesions are rare in oriental and almost unknown
                  in black races. They typically occur in 'sun-
                  worshipping' blonde subjects and on the exposed
                  skin of outdoor workers.

83 A **True**   they are raised, reddish-purple dermal vascular
   B **False**   malformations. They have no malignant potential.
   C **False**   the vast majority will spontaneously regress by 3
   D **False**   years of age. If this does not occur then a short dose of
                  steroids may initiate regression. Radiotherapy for this
                  or any other benign lesion is to be condemned
                  because of the possible dangers of ensuing
                  malignancies. Surgery is rarely necessary. Capillary
                  angiomas should be distinguished from cavernous
                  angiomas which develop from larger vessels. The
                  latter appear in childhood, do not regress and
                  frequently require surgical treatment.

84 A **True**   the peak incidence is in the third decade.
   B **False**   they are firm, smooth, well circumscribed, mobile
                  lumps.
   C **True**   in the majority of patients this is so.
   D **False**   they tend to enlarge.

85   Fibrocystic disease of the breast
    A   is a variant of the normal cyclical changes that the breast
         undergoes during menstruation
    B   is normally unilateral
    C   tends to progress in the post-menopausal years
    D   is precancerous

86   The management of fibrocystic breast disease should
    A   usually be by surgical excision
    B   include mammography when available
    C   include therapy with oestrogens
    D   include therapy with progesterone

87   An intraduct papilloma of the breast
    A   may cause a bloody nipple discharge
    B   may be diagnosed with the aid of contrast radiography
    C   should be treated by simple mastectomy
    D   is associated with fibrocystic disease of the breast

88   Paget's disease of the nipple
    A   usually presents as a bilateral eczema of the nipple
    B   is always related to an underlying breast cancer
    C   indicates incurable breast cancer
    D   has non-specific histological characteristics

85 A **True**   there is glandular hyperplasia, cyst formation, duct
                   wall hyperplasia, periductal fibrosis and lymphocytic
                   infiltration.
   B **False**   it is usually bilateral and most common in the upper
                   outer quadrant of the breasts.
   C **False**   though it is most common in the later years of
                   reproductive life, some regression and decrease in
                   pain occurs after the menopause.
   D **False**   there is no conclusive evidence to support this view.

86 A **False**   this is an extremely common condition and the
                   majority of patients are treated symptomatically. Only
                   when the lesion is discrete and carcinoma is
                   suspected is an excision biopsy undertaken.
   B **True**   where this facility exists, advantage should be taken
                   of its ability to distinguish breast cancer from
                   fibrocystic disease. It may also detect a neoplasm
                   whose diagnosis is obscured by surrounding (and
                   unrelated) fibrocystic disease of the breast.
   C **False**   these do not influence the progress of the disease
   D **False**   although some pain relief may be achieved.

87 A **True**   this and the occurrence of pain are the most frequent
                   symptoms.
   B **True**   injection of the relevant duct with contrast medium
                   often confirms the diagnosis.
   C **False**   local removal of this benign lesion with or without
                   segmental resection of the breast is all that is required.
   D **False**   this benign neoplasm is not to be confused with the
                   diffuse papillomatous lesions often seen in fibrocystic
                   breast disease.

88 A **False**   it is usually a unilateral disease.
   B **True**   the lesion is an intraduct carcinoma arising in the
                   minute ducts of the nipple. It infiltrates the skin and
                   often extends deeply to produce a palpable mass.
   C **False**   there is a good prognosis in these tumours
                   compared to other breast cancers. This is probably
                   related to earlier diagnosis and treatment.
   D **False**   the histology is characteristic, viz: large clear
                   vacuolated cells (Paget's cells) invading the dermis,
                   epidermal hypertrophy and dermal lymphocytic
                   infiltration

89   X-ray examination of the breast (mammography)
  A does not improve the clinician's diagnosis rate of benign and malignant breast disease
  B is diagnostically most useful in young women
  C is practical as a nationwide presymptomatic screening procedure in the United Kingdom
  D contributes nothing to the management of the patients with clinically obvious breast cancer

90   Breast cancer
  A is the commonest female neoplasm in the United Kingdom
  B has its highest incidence in social class V
  C has a familial tendency
  D is less common in nulliparous women

91   Breast cancer
  A often presents with a history of breast pain
  B is most common in the upper outer quadrant of the breast
  C can be diagnosed preoperatively by the experienced clinician in 95 per cent of cases
  D must be considered on discovering any discrete mass in the breast

92   The signs and symptoms of breast cancer include
  A a milky nipple discharge
  B eczematous changes in the nipple and areola
  C pre-menstrual breast pain
  D skin tethering

89 A **False**   the diagnosis rate is improved by 10 to 15 per cent.
    B **False**   the active young breast is relatively radio-opaque and the infiltrating opacification and punctate calcification of breast cancer are rendered more difficult to see.
    C **False**   the logistic demands of this screening technique, in terms of manpower and equipment, are far too excessive.
    D **False**   mammography may reveal impalpable cancers and thus bilateral cancers will be diagnosed twice as frequently.

90 A **True**   followed by large bowel and uterine cancer.
    B **False**   the highest incidence is in social class 1.
    C **True**   a maternal history or a history of a sibling with the disease increases the incidence of breast cancer up to 15 times that of the general population.
    D **False**   nulliparous women have the highest incidence of breast cancer, followed by those who did not have their first child until 25 years of age. Breast feeding seems to confer some slight protection.

91 A **True**   though a painless lump is the first sign in two-thirds of patients, in more than 15 per cent pain is the presenting symptom.
    B **True**   half the breast cancer occurs in the upper outer quadrant and only 5 per cent in the lower inner quadrant. Medial lesions are much less common.
    C **False**   most studies show clinical diagnosis to be accurate in only 70 per cent of cases — thus all discrete non-cystic breast lumps must be subjected to biopsy.
    D **True**

92 A **False**   cancer should be suspected if a nipple discharge is bloodstained.
    B **True**   Paget's disease of the nipple, which produces eczematous changes in the nipple, is always associated with an underlying breast cancer.
    C **False**   this usually indicates fibrocystic disease of the breast.
    D **True**   this is best observed in the skin directly over the tumour. Apart from cancer only acute inflammation and fat necrosis show this sign.

93   The histological study of breast cancers has shown that
  A the prognosis is not related to histological type
  B the commonest carcinoma is a squamous carcinoma
  C most breast cancers arise from the epithelium of the breast lobule
  D satellite breast cancers are common

94   Signs of incurable breast cancer include
  A tumour fixity to the chest wall
  B skin ulceration
  C Palpably enlarged mobile ipsilateral axillary lymph nodes
  D a bloody nipple discharge

95   The incidence of breast cancer
  A increases with age
  B decreases after premenopausal oophorectomy
  C is relatively low in Japan
  D is related to uterine cancer

96   In a patient with breast neoplasia distant metastases may be revealed by
  A a radiographic skeletal survey
  B a raised serum alkaline phosphatase
  C raised urinary 17-Ketosteroid metabolites
  D a raised serum glutamic oxaloacetic transminase (SGOT)

93 A **False**   study of untreated patients with breast cancer reveals that the prognosis is related to the histological type. The medullary carcinoma, which is least invasive, has the best prognosis.
  B **False**   the vast majority are adenocarcinomata.
  C **True**   breast cancers arise from the nipple, the ducts or the lobule epithelium. Duct cancer is by far the commonest.
  D **True**   this is well marked in the commonest tumour—the infiltrating adenocarcinoma (scirrhous carcinoma) where early invasion of blood and lymph vessels occurs.

94 A **True**   these two signs together with peau d'orange,
  B **True**   lymphoedema of the arm and fixed axillary lymph nodes usually indicate incurable advanced cancer of the breast.
  C **False**   more than half the enlarged axillary nodes associated with a breast neoplasm contain no tumour. This may be the result of an immune response to the tumour.
  D **False**   a bloody discharge may indicate ductal cancer, or invasion of a major duct by cancer but it need not indicate advanced or incurable disease.

95 A **True**   there is an increasing incidence with age after puberty.
  B **True**   oophorectomy before 40 years of age considerably reduces the expected incidence.
  C **True**   the incidence in Japan is less than 20 per cent of that in Britain and the USA.
  D **False**   no causal or associated relationship has been shown to exist.

96 A **True**   although almost half the patients presenting with
  B **True**   breast cancer have occult, and at present mostly
  C **False**   unidentifiable, metastatic deposits, a careful clinical
  D **True**   examination and some routine investigations will reveal some of these deposits. A chest X-ray and a skeletal survey will reveal some of the chest and bone secondaries, and the serum alkaline phosphatase and SGOT may be elevated with liver deposits. No serum urinary factor at present estimated is diagnostic of widespread disease. It is debatable whether radioisotope scanning of the bones and liver are justifiable as a routine measure as yet because of their diagnostic limitations.

97   Palliation of advanced incurable breast cancer
   A   can be achieved by therapy with anti-oestrogens.
   B   can be achieved by oestrogen administration in the
        premenopausal patient
   C   can be achieved by androgen administration in the
        postmenopausal patient
   D   can be achieved by chemotherapeutic agents in pre- and post
        menopausal patients

98   The prognosis of treated breast cancer
   A   is related to the clinical staging of the cancer
   B   is related to the number of axillary nodes found to be invaded
        by cancer at operation
   C   is related to the use of postoperative radiotherapy to the
        regional nodes and operative field
   D   is better after simple rather than radical mastectomy

99   The prognosis of treated Stage 1 breast cancer
   A   cannot be satisfactorily assessed until 15 years have elapsed
   B   is adversely affected by a subsequent pregnancy
   C   is worse in the male
   D   is worse if the cancer is discovered during late pregnancy or
        the puerperium

50% 22/2/91
72% 18/3

97 A **True**   this should be the first procedure to be
               tried — approximately one-third of patients will
               respond.
    B **False**   in this group oestrogens often have a stimulatory
               effect on the cancer. Oestrogen-containing
               contraceptive pills are thus contra-indicated.
    C **True**   about 20 per cent of patients will respond.
    D **True**   single agents such as 5-Fluorouracil and quadruple
               chemotherapy with added cyclophosphamide,
               vincristine and methotrexate have been shown to
               produce moderately high remission rates in both
               groups of patients.

98 A **True**   when treated, approximately 65 per cent of patients
               with Stage 1 (Manchester Classification) are alive after
               5 years, whereas survival rates of Stage II, III and IV
               are progressively worse.
    B **True**   when only 2 or 3 nodes are found to contain tumour
               and these are removed, survival rates approach those
               of Stage 1. More than 4 affected nodes worsens the
               prognosis considerably.
    C **False**   no improvement in longevity following regional
               radiotherapy as an adjuvant to surgery has been
               found in patients with breast cancer. Local recurrence
               of the disease is however diminished.
    D **False**   survival and recurrence rates appear to be similar in
               the various methods of treatment of 'operable' breast
               cancer. This similarity reflects the inadequacies of
               clinical staging in that the consequences of occult,
               unidentified metastases may disguise the small
               differences between the various methods of
               treatment.

99 A **True**   the vast majority of recurrent breast neoplasms occur
               in the first 15 years after treatment. Survival rate after
               15 years parallels that of a comparable age group in
               the general population.
    B **False**   the survival rate is significantly improved in those
               patients who become pregnant after treatment for
               breast cancer (although oestrogens have a deleterious
               effects in advanced breast neoplasia in this age group).
    C **False**   stage for stage, survival rates are similar in the two
               sexes, but early spread to adjoining tissues renders
               more male breast cancers surgically incurable.
    D **True**   the survival rate is about 5 per cent below that of
               matched groups of non-pregnant patients.

6 Thyroid, Parathyroid and Adrenal Glands

100 Signs and symptoms of hyperthyroidism include
- A decreased sweating
- B an irregular pulse rate
- C cardiac failure
- D diplopia

101 Symptoms of hyperthyroidism include
- A intolerance to cold
- B increased appetite
- C emotional instability
- D diarrhoea

102 Medical therapy of hyperthyroidism
- A is particularly indicated in the pregnant patient
- B will usually produce a long-lasting remission rate of 70 to 80 per cent after a 6-month course
- C is occasionally complicated by bone marrow depression
- D depends on the efficacy of the drugs in inhibiting the hypothalamic centres which govern thyroid stimulating hormone (TSH) release by the pituitary

103 Treatment of hyperthyroidism with radioactive iodine
- A is complicated by the late occurrence of thyroid cancer
- B should not be undertaken in patients below the age of 40
- C is frequently complicated by the development of myxoedema
- D is often complicated by a short-lived exacerbation of the hyperthyroid state

100 A **False**   there is increased sweating, producing the
                     characteristic warm sweaty palms of the thyrotoxic
                     patient.
     B **True**   atrial fibrillation is particularly common in the elderly
     C **True**   and the deleterious effects on the cardiac output may
                     produce cardiac failure in this group of patients.
     D **True**   multiple eye signs of this condition include
                     exophthalmos, lid lag and opthalmoplegia, producing
                     the characteristic facies of the severely thyrotoxic
                     patient.

101 A **False**   amongst the host of symptoms, the most
     B **True**   characteristic are weight loss associated with an
     C **True**   increased appetite. There is marked heat intolerance
     D **True**   and the development of irritability and emotional
                     instability. Diarrhoea and dysmenorrhoea may be
                     prominent.

102 A **False**   these drugs may cross the placental barrier and inhibit
                     fetal thyroid function. They may also be excreted in
                     breast milk.
     B **False**   recurrence of hyperthyroidism after drug withdrawal
                     occurs in up to 70 per cent of patients.
     C **True**   both propylthiouracil and carbimazole produce
                     agranulocytosis in a small number of patients. Drug
                     rashes and hepatitis also occur.
     D **False**   the thiouracil group of drugs acts by interfering with
                     the organic binding of iodine; carbimazole by
                     interfering with tri-iodothyronine synthesis in the
                     gland.

103 A **False**   cumulative experience and close study of patients in
     B **True**   the 25 years since the introduction of therapy with
                     radioactive iodine reveals no increased risk of
                     neoplasia. It is advisable however to restrict its use to
                     those patients in the latter half of life.
     C **True**   this may not develop for several years after treatment
                     and the incidence of hypothyroidism seems to vary in
                     different centres. Hypothyroidism rates of 40 per cent
                     10 years after treatment are common and this fraction
                     appears to increase with the passage of time.
     D **False**   the treatment has no stimulant effect on the gland. Its
                     beneficial effects are not usually seen for a month or
                     two after ingestion of the radioactive iodine.

104   The surgical treatment of hyperthyroidism
  A   is commonly followed by hypothyroidism
  B   has a high rate of recurrence
  C   can be safely effected without preoperative drug therapy
  D   may be complicated by postoperative high parathormone
      levels

105   A multinodular (adenomatous) qoitre
  A   is more common in those patients having a deficient
      iodine intake
  B   is usually preceded by a diffuse goitre in early adult life
  C   is usually a precancerous condition
  D   is effectively treated with thyroid hormones to prevent
      further adenomatous changes

106   Auto-immune thyroiditis (Hashimoto's disease)
  A   characteristically occurs in young females
  B   often presents with hyperthyroidism
  C   produces a soft diffuse enlargement of the thyroid gland
  D   is associated with regional lymph node enlargement

104 A **False**   postoperative hypothyroidism can be detected in 5 to
    B **False**   10 per cent of patients. There is a similar incidence of
                  recurrent thyrotoxicosis.
    C **False**   to operate on the hyperthyroid gland is to court the
                  life-threatening condition of 'thyroid crisis' — acute
                  severe hyperthyroidism. The patient must be
                  rendered euthyroid preoperatively with antithyroid
                  drugs and/or beta-blockers such as propanolol.
    D **False**   postoperative hypoparathyroidism occurs in a small
                  proportion of patients either due to disturbance to the
                  blood supply of the parathyroids or their inadvertent
                  removal.

105 A **True**   this has given rise to the term 'endemic goitre' for it
                  refers to the high incidence of multinodular goitre in
                  those areas low in naturally occurring iodine, e.g.
                  Derbyshire in the United Kingdom, Switzerland and
                  the Andes.
    B **True**   TSH stimulation, secondary to the iodine deficiency,
                  results initially in diffuse hyperplasia. This is followed
                  years later by the development of nodules of
                  hyperplastic gland interposed with areas of involution
                  and fibrosis.
    C **False**   although the incidence of thyroid cancer is increased
                  in some areas of endemic goitre there is no evidence
                  to suggest a direct relationship between multinodular
                  goitre and neoplasia in the United Kingdom.
    D **True**   thyroid hormone administration suppresses the effect
                  of TSH on the adenomatous gland. In the early stages
                  of the disease iodine can halt the development of a
                  multinodular goitre from diffuse glandular
                  enlargement.

106 A **False**   it occurs most frequently in middle aged females.
    B **True**   this is usually mild and short lived and is followed by
                  the development of permanent hypothyroidism.
    C **False**   diffuse enlargement of the gland does occur, but the
                  gland is firm and rubbery.
    D **False**   lymphadenopathy is not a feature of Hashimoto's
                  disease and if present should arouse suspicion of
                  thyroid neoplasia.

107   Hashimoto's disease
    A is often associated with increased levels of circulating thyroid antibodies
    B is characterised by lymphocytic infiltration and fibrosis of the thyroid gland
    C is usually treated by sub-total thyroidectomy
    D should be treated by anti-thyroid drugs

108   Thyroid cancer
    A frequently produces multinodular enlargement of the gland
    B should be diagnosed by preoperative needle biopsy of the gland
    C can be excluded if there is a localised but soft enlargement of the gland
    D often produces a bruit over the gland

109   Papillary carcinoma of the thyroid
    A may follow radiation exposure in childhood
    B is a slow growing tumour
    C usually metastasises to lymph nodes
    D is usually a multifocal tumour

110   Follicular carcinoma of the thyroid
    A is most common in females
    B is most common above the age of 30 years
    C usually metastasises to lymph nodes
    D is associated with a relatively good prognosis in childhood

111   Undifferentiated carcinoma of the thyroid
    A is most common in females
    B is most common above the age of 60
    C is often thyroid stimulating hormone (TSH) dependent
    D often exhibits independent thyroid hormone production

107 A **True**   there is often a raised titre of anti-thyroglobulin
                    antibodies and antibodies against thyroid acinar cells.
     B **True**   fibrosis is a manifestation of the later stages of the
                    disease.
     C **False**   the appropriate treatment is very individual. It is
     D **True**   advisable to take an open thyroid biopsy; pressure on
                    the trachea may demand excision of the thyroid
                    isthmus and very occasionally cosmetic
                    considerations require a sub-total thyroidectomy.
                    Thyroid hormones usually have to be given to combat
                    hypothyroidism.

108 A **False**   whilst cancer occasionally develops in a multinodular
                    goitre the usual signs of thyroid neoplasia are a
                    localised or generalised swelling of the gland.
     B **False**   it is difficult to diagnose well-differentiated cancers
                    from the small piece of tissue so obtained and spread
                    of cancer along the needle track occasionally occurs.
     C **False**   well-differentiated lesions frequently present as soft
                    solitary swellings. All solitary swellings of the gland
                    should have an excision biopsy performed.
     D **False**   there is no hypervascularity in thyroid cancer.

109 A **True**   this is most marked in cancers appearing before
                    adolescence. A history of irradiation has been noted in
                    70 per cent of papillary cancers in this age group.
     B **True**   this is particularly so in young patients where growth
                    of the primary and metastases is slow.
     C **True**   whilst this is the most common mode of spread,
                    spread by the blood stream is not uncommon in the
                    older patient.
     D **True**   this is frequently noted and may represent
                    intraglandular spread.

110 A **True**   as is papillary carcinoma.
     B **True**   whereas papillary carcinoma is most common in
                    children and younger adults.
     C **False**   though lymphatic spread does occur, spread by the
                    blood stream to bones and lungs is more frequent.
     D **True**   there is an increased incidence of well-differentiated,
                    well-encapsulated follicular and papillary carcinomas
                    in this age group and they are associated with good
                    prognosis.

111 A **False**   there is an equal incidence in the two sexes.
     B **True**   it rarely occurs before this age.
     C **False**   the histological picture is of sheets of undifferentiated
     D **False**   cells with no follicular formation. No evidence of
                    hormonal activity or response to hormonal therapy
                    exists in this type of tumour.

112   The surgical treatment of thyroid cancer
    A   should be by 'near total' thyroidectomy in the potentially
         curable patient
    B   should include block dissection of the neighbouring lymph
         nodes whether or not they appear to contain tumour
    C   is most successful in the papillary type of cancer
    D   should be preceded by a therapeutic dose of 1^{131}

113   Recurrent thyroid cancer can effectively be treated by
    A   high doses of 1^{131}
    B   high doses of thyroid hormone
    C   external irradiation
    D   chemotherapy

114   The earliest symptoms of hyperparathyroidism include
    A   diarrhoea
    B   polydipsia and polyuria
    C   unexplained weight gain
    D   muscle spasm

115   Primary hyperparathyroidism
    A   is most common in postmenopausal females
    B   is occasionally diagnosed by routine biochemical screening
         of patients
    C   should be considered when a patient presents with tetany
    D   can be caused by adenomas or hyperplasia of the glands

112 A **True** many of the tumours are multifocal and only the posterior rim of thyroid tissue (and associated parathyroid glands) on the opposite side of the neck to the primary tumour should be preserved.
     B **False** only node dissection of apparently involved nodes should be attempted.
     C **True** the histological type and the presence or absence of invasion are of great significance in determining the outcome after surgical treatment. Long term survival has been frequently recorded in incompletely removed papillary and follicular corcinomata of the thyroid where these are well differentiated, whereas undifferentiated cancers are uniformly fatal whatever the treatment.
     D **False** histological diagnosis may be interfered with. I^{131} has no part to play in preoperative therapy.

113 A **True** a therapeutic dose of radioactive iodine is the
     B **True** treatment of choice. TSH suppression by means of
     C **True** thyroid hormones is used in well-differentiated
     D **False** tumours with good results. External irradiation is of value in palliating undifferentiated tumours and lymphomas. There are as yet no reports of satisfactory remission rates being produced by chemotherapy.

114 A **False** the earliest symtoms are vague and rarely suggest the
     B **True** diagnosis but constipation, muscle weakness,
     C **False** anorexia and weight loss together with thirst and
     D **False** polyuria are encountered.

115 A **True** it is three times more common in females and particularly frequent between 45 and 65 years of age. It is rare in children.
     B **True** the rate of recognition has increased since
     C **False** biochemical screening has been introduced. A raised
     D **True** serum calcium, particularly if associated with a low serum phosphate, is a strong pointer to the diagnosis. tetany only occurs with a low serum calcium. The commonest presenting symptoms are vague abdominal and bone pains. Fractures are not uncommon and renal calculi may produce renal or ureteric colic. Thus the adage; hyperparathyroidism equals 'groans, bones and stones'.
single adenomata are the most common cause of the condition. Generalised hyperplasia may cause hyperparathyroidism. Carcinoma is very rarely encountered.

116   Skeletal signs, symptoms and radiological evidence of hyperparathyroidism
A   include demineralisation of the bones
B   include bone cysts and osteoclastoma formation
C   include spontaneous fractures
D   are the most common presenting complaints

117   Renal symptoms of hyperparathyroidism
A   may be due to renal stones
B   may be due to nephrocalcinosis
C   are frequently those of chronic renal failure
D   are associated with hypertension

118   Acute adrenal insufficiency
A   in the newborn is due to haemorrhage into one or both adrenal glands
B   in the newborn typically occurs in the second week of life
C   in the adult usually follows a pneumococcal septicaemia
D   in the adult is most frequently encountered following bilateral adrenalectomy

119   Phaeochromocytomas
A   are tumours of the spinal nerve roots
B   are frequently multiple
C   characteristically present with a lemon-yellow skin discolouration
D   can be effectively managed by long term medical therapy

116 A **True**   this is a general phenomenon affecting the whole skeleton.
    B **True**   this is particularly common in the bones of the lower limbs and ribs.
    C **True**   these indicate advanced and severe hyperparathyroidism.
    D **False**   the most common presenting signs and symtoms are those referrable to the renal tract.

117 A **True**   renal stones occur in over half the patients.
    B **True**   nephrocalcinosis is less common, about 5 per cent of patients being affected.
    C **True**   more than 70 per cent of patients have renal damage and this may be severe especially when nephrocalcinosis is present.
    D **True**   more than 70 per cent of patients have hypertension and in the majority this is associated with renal damage.

118 A **True**   adrenal apoplexy in the newborn is usually fatal
    B **False**   within the first few days of life. Haemorrhage into the glands occurs at birth and is possibly precipitated by withdrawal of maternal hormones. The condition is sometimes associated with birth trauma.
    C **False**   while streptococcal, staphylococcal and pneumococcal septicaemia may all give rise to the Waterhouse-Friderichsen syndrome it is most commonly associated with fulminating meningococcal septicaemia.
    D **False**   this should be prevented by the routine administration of steroid replacement during and after the operation.

119 A **False**   they arise from chromaffin cells of the adrenal medulla and sympathetic nervous system.
    B **True**   40 per cent are multiple.
    C **False**   the characteristic symptoms are due to intermittent
    D **False**   catecholamine release and thus all the symptoms and signs of sympathetic overactivity such as paroxysmal tachycardia, flushing, sweating and palpitations are intermittently produced. Hypertension will eventually become permanent and diabetes is often present.
                  prompt surgical treatment is the rule. During the operation undue handling of the tumour may result in a very serious tachycardia and a dangerous attack of hypertension. These problems are reduced by effective preoperative sympathetic blockade.

120   In Cushing's syndrome
    A   there is usually an increased deposition of fat over the face
        and trunk
    B   hypotension and hypokalaemia are frequently present
    C   there is an increased production of adrenal hormones
    D   the cause is most frequently an adrenal tumour

121   Cushing's syndrome
    A   may be due to adrenal cortical hyperplasia, adrenal
        adenomata or adrenal carcinomata
    B   may be associated with bronchogenic cancer
    C   is effectively treated by total bilateral adrenalectomy even
        when shown to be pituitary dependent
    D   should be managed medically unless complications develop

122   A thyroglossal cyst
    A   usually presents in early adult life
    B   is a remnant of fifth pharyngeal arch mesoderm
    C   should usually be excised with the thyroid cartilage
    D   does not move with swallowing

120 A **True**   facial and truncal adiposity, polycythaemia, diabetes
and skin striae are characteristic findings. The serum
potassium is invariably high and hypertension is
common.
   B **False**   diagnostic confirmation can be obtained by serum
   C **True**   estimations and urinalysis.
   D **False**   more than half the cases studied show the causative
lesion to be in the pituitary. This liberates ACTH and
stimulates the adrenals into overactivity.

121 A **True**   these account for approximately half of the patients
seen; the remainder are secondary to pituitary
overactivity and a few other rare causes (see B).
   B **True**   ectopic ACTH may be produced by several neoplasms·
of which lung is the commonest.
   C **True**   this is usually successful. There is a high rate of
recurrence if a subtotal adrenalectomy is performed.
   D **False**   there is, as yet, no curative medical treatment and
since the patient progressively worsens, surgical
treatment is always advised.

122 A **False**   they most frequently appear before adulthood and
one-third of them appear before the age of 10 years.
   B **False**   the thyroid develops as a downgrowth from the back
of the tongue into the third and fourth pharyngeal
arches. A thyroglossal cyst is a remnant along the
course of this tract.
   C **False**   but it is usually necessary to remove the body of the
hyoid bone in order to follow, and remove, the tract
into the base of the tongue.
   D **False**   like the thyroid gland it moves with the larynx in
swallowing.

123 Neuroblastomata
    A usually arise in the renal substance
    B are one of the rarest solid tumours of childhood
    C usually metastasise via the blood stream
    D are difficult to distinguish from Wilms' tumours on clinical
        examination

124 Neuroblastomata
    A characteristically produce 5-hydroxyindole acetic acid which
        can be detected in the urine
    B rarely metastasise to bone
    C cannot be satisfactorily treated by surgery
    D have a better porgnosis in younger patients

123 A **False**   these are malignancies of the primitive cells of the
sympathetic nervous system, consequently they most
frequently arise in the adrenals and less commonly in
the sympathetic chain.
   B **False**   they are the commonest solid tumour of infancy.
   C **True**   this is common and spread to lungs and bones is
frequently seen; local lymphatic spread is also usually
present.
   D **False**   their nodularity and fixity, especially during
respiration, usually enable this distinction to be made.

124 A **False**   most tumours secrete detectable amounts of
noradrenaline precursors, e.g. 3-methoxy-4-mandelic
acid (VMA).
   B **False**   bone deposits are found in 30 to 40 per cent of
patients.
   C **False**   radical surgery is the basis of treatment. In recent
   D **True**   years postoperative radiotherapy and routine use of
vincristine and cyclophosphamide have each been
shown to improve survival rates. Spontaneous
regression of metastases occasionally occurs. Cure
rates of 25 per cent for abdominal neuroblastomata
and of 50 per cent (if the child is less than 1 year old)
have been reported.

7 Oral Cavity, Pharynx and Oesophagus

125 Surgical repair of a cleft lip and palate
A should not be undertaken until the child begins to talk
B is essential for normal feeding of the child
C is essential to ensure normal development of speech
D should frequently be combined with dental prosthetic work

126 Salivary duct calculi
A produce pain on eating
B are commonest in the parotid ducts
C are a common cause of acute parotitis
D are associated with hypercalcaemic states

127 Salivary tumours
A occur most commonly in the parotid gland
B of the parotid gland producing facial nerve lesions
are usually malignant
C may appear as palatal swellings
D are in most cases satisfactorily treated by radiotherapy

128 Cancer of the tongue
A is usually an adenocarcinoma
B is more common in males
C most commonly presents as an indolent ulcer
D metastasises via the lymphatics at an early stage of the
disease

125 A ~~True~~ *False*   early closure of the defects is desirable whatever their
     B True   form; cleft lips at about 3 months and palates at 9–12
     C True   months. In this way suckling difficulties are overcome,
                  there is a likelihood of normal voice development and
                  cosmetic deformities are minimised.
     D True   bilateral palatal clefts often require staged surgical
                  correction and an occlusive dental palatal plate may
                  allow normal voice development.

126 A True   the increased production of salivary juice produces
                  painful distension of the gland.
     B False   the submandibular salivary duct is far more
                  commonly affected.
     C False   the common causes of acute parotitis are debility,
                  dehydration and poor oral hygiene.
     D False   there is no evidence that generalised metabolic
                  disorders play any part in the formation of salivary
                  duct calculi. Their aetiology is obscure but may be
                  related to a disturbance in the pH of the saliva.

127 A True   75 per cent of all salivary gland tumours occur in the
                  parotid.
     B True   the majority of parotid tumours are benign (and of
                  these, the commonest is the mixed parotid tumour)
                  but malignancy is likely if there is an associated facial
                  nerve palsy, an infiltration of the overlying skin or
                  cervical lymph node enlargement.
     C True   the small and numerous salivary glands of the palate
                  may become neoplastic — the commonest tumour
                  being the highly malignant cylindroma.
     D False   surgical excision is the basis of treatment — together
                  with removal of any associated involved nodes.

128 A False   though adenocarcinomas do occur, more than 95 per
     B True   cent of tongue cancers are of squamous origin
                  it occurs four times as frequently in males. There is
                  often a history of chronic irritation, leukoplakia,
                  chronic alcoholism or long-standing iron deficiency
                  anaemia.
     C True   infiltrative forms of the cancer are recognised but the
                  commonest presentation is of a chronic painless ulcer.
     D True   more than half the patients have lymph node deposits
                  at the time of presentation and, with cancers of the
                  dorsum of the tongue, these may be bilateral. Surgical
                  excision of the primary tumour and affected lymph
                  nodes forms the basis of treatment. On occasions this
                  is supplemented with radiotherapy.

129 Pharyngeal pouches
A usually occur at the pharyngo-oesophageal junction
B are commonest in young people
C may cause pulmonary problems
D usually require surgical excision

130 Pharyngo-oesophageal diverticula
A only occur at the level of cricopharyngeus
B may be related to para-oesophageal lymph nodes
C are often associated with recurrent attacks of pneumonitis
D characteristically present with vomiting

131 The diagnosis of oesophageal achalasia may be made by
A oesophageal biopsy
B barium swallow X-ray examination
C oesophagoscopy
D oesophageal motility studies

132 In oesophageal achalasia
A dysphagia is usually the first symptom
B pain is rarely a prominent symptom
C there is an absence of peristalsis in the oesophagus
D there is an absence of ganglion cells in Auerbach's plexus in the wall of the oesophagus ·

129 A **False** the commonest site is to the left of the midline
posteriorly, between the oblique fibres and the
transverse cricopharyngeal portion of the inferior
constrictor muscle of the pharynx.
B **False** the majority occur in elderly patients.
C **True** aspiration of the diverticular contents may occur,
particularly at night, producing aspiration
pneumonitis. In addition, dysphagia and gurgling
during deglutition may be present.
D **True** excision of the diverticulum and closure of the
pharyngeal wall is the usual method of treatment.

130 A **False** there are three common sites of occurrence, at the
B **True** level of cricopharyngeus, just above the diaphragm,
and in the mid-oesophageal region.
C **True** aspiration of oesophageal contents is a consequence
of the larger diverticula. This occurs particularly at
night.
D **False** regurgitation, noisy eating and dysphagia are the
commonest symptoms.

131 A **False** the neurological changes lie submucosally and a deep
biopsy would be needed. This is a dangerous
procedure.
B **True** the characteristic finding is of a dilated oesophagus
norrowing down in a conical fashion to a smooth
stenosis of the cardia.
C **True** this will distinguish early achalasia from a benign
stricture or cancer.
D **True** in advanced cases there is no peristalsis and no
swallowing reflex present. The oesophagus empties
purely by gravity.

132 A **True** this is often more marked for liquids than solids, and
is eased by 'trick' swallowing manoeuvres by the
patient.
B **False** in more than 25 per cent of cases the patient
complains of diffuse retrosternal pain in the early
stages of the disease. This decreases as the functional
obstruction worsens.
C **True** the oesophagus is immobile, dilated and empties only
by gravity through a lower oesophageal sphincter
which does not relax (cardiospasm).
D **True** whether this is a primary or secondary phenomenon
is not known, but it is present in the majority of cases.

133   The treatment of oesophageal achalasia
   A   is usually by a cardiomyotomy (Heller's operation)
   B   should primarily be by dilatation
   C   should be by oesophagogastrectomy
   D   should include a transthoracic vagotomy

134   'Sideropaenic dysphagia'
   A   is associated with koilonychia and atrophic oral mucosa
   B   is related to longstanding Vitamin B_{12} deficiency
   C   is also known eponymously as the 'Paterson-Kelly syndrome'
        or the 'Plummer-Vinson syndrome'
   D   is usually due to an oesophageal cancer

135   Sliding hiatus herniae
   A   are associated with a dilated diaphragmatic hiatus
   B   are usually readily reducible
   C   are usually asymptomatic
   D   occasionally strangulate

136   The symptoms of peptic oesophagitis
   A   include intermittent dysphagia
   B   are often associated with those of anaemia
   C   include retrosternal discomfort
   D   are more likely to occur when the patient is in the upright
        position

133 A **True**   the vast majority of patients are helped by this procedure though postoperative reflux oesophagitis may occasionally be a problem.

   B **False**   early cases can be dealt with in this way. Oesophageal perforation is an occasional complication of this procedure.

   C **False**   this is too extensive a procedure and is not rational since the stomach is free of any pathology.

   D **False**   section of the vagus has no effect on oesophageal motility.

134 A **True**   the majority of cases occur in middle aged or elderly women.

   B **False**   the majority of cases are associated with long-standing iron deficiency anaemia. The reason for this association is obscure.

   C **True**   it was first described in 1919 by Paterson and Kelly.

   D **False**   the commonest cause is a fibrous web occuring in the upper oesophagus. However, about 10 per cent of patients develop cancers of the oesophagus, pharynx or oral cavity.

135 A **True**   the cardiac portion of the stomach herniates into the mediastinum through a dilated hiatus.

   B **True**   the oesophagogastric junction will return to the abdomen very readily unless oesophageal ulceration or stricture has resulted in shortening of the oesophagus.

   C **True**   incidental asymptomatic sliding hiatus herniae are frequently demonstrated by radiologists.

   D **False**   these herniae, though not always reducible, have a wide neck at the diaphragmatic hiatus and do not strangulate.

136 A **True**   severe oesophagitis produces mucosal oedema and spasm of the underlying oesophageal muscle. This is often intermittent. Submucosal inflammatory changes may eventually produce fibrosis and a stricture of the lower end of the oesophagus. This is often associated with an alleviation of the symptoms of oesophagitis since reflux occurs less readily through the stricture.

   B **True**   chronic blood loss may occur from the inflamed and haemorrhagic oesophageal mucosa.

   C **True**   retrosternal discomfort is the commonest symptom but discomfort also may be produced in the neck, chest and epigastrium.

   D **False**   this position often relieves the discomfort, which is usually produced by stooping and lying down.

137   Peptic oesophagitis
   A   is effectively demonstrated by a barium swallow and meal
   B   can be readily confirmed by oesophagoscopy
   C   is associated with the production of higher than normal
        amounts of gastric acid
   D   is a condition confined to adults

138   The successful medical management of peptic oesophagitis
   A   should include anticholinergic drugs
   B   includes weight reduction
   C   includes elevating the head of the bed
   D   depends on regular antacid administration

139   Surgical management of peptic oesophagitis
   A   is indicated in the majority of patients
   B   is based on the prevention of reflux
   C   is best restricted to repeated bouginage when peptic
        stricture are present
   D   should include a vagotomy

137 A **False** though radiologists are often successful at demonstrating a sliding hiatus hernia, it is known that only some of these patients will have oesophagitis. Oesophagitis may also occur without a hernia being demonstrated. The radiological demonstration of oesophagitis is not usually possible unless spasm or stenosis exists.

B **True** this is the most important investigation. The inflamed mucosa can be recognised by its friability and by contact bleeding. Occasionally ulceration of the mucosa will be seen.

C **False** no relationship between acid output and oesophagitis has been demonstrated. It may be that bile salts are the noxious constituents of the fluid reflux. There is no association with duodenal ulceration.

D **False** infants born with a congenital hiatus hernia suffer from reflux and oesophagitis.

138 A **False** these are not helpful.

B **True** weight reduction may reduce intra-abdominal

C **True** pressure but it only alleviates the symptoms slightly. Elevation of the head of the bed is worthwhile, especially in patients with mild symptoms. Regular small meals and reduction in smoking are also of benefit.

D **True** they provide symptomatic relief and may reduce reflux by increasing the tone of the gastro-oesophageal sphincter.

139 A **False** the necessary surgical procedure involves a major abdominal or thoracic operation. It has a significant morbidity and a small mortality. Only incapacitating symptoms are an indication for surgery.

B **True** several surgical procedures exist and their rationale is, in all cases, the prevention of reflux.

C **False** bouginage will provide only short term relief. It permits reflux to recur with the recurrence of oesophagitis. Bouginage combined with surgical prevention of reflux is, however, very satisfactory management.

D **False** reducing gastric acid secretion has a minimal effect on oesophagitis.

140   Para-oesophageal hiatus herniae
   A   usually occur through a defect in the diaphragm to the right of
      the oesophagus
   B   usually have an easily recognised hernial sac
   C   are usually accompanied by oesophagitis
   D   may produce postprandial chest pain

141   Para-oesophageal hiatus herniae
   A   are frequently associated with gastric ulceration
   B   are frequently accompanied by occult gastrointestinal blood
      loss
   C   are congenital in origin
   D   should be managed conservatively in the majority of patients

142   Cancer of the oesophagus
   A   usually presents with intermittent dysphagia
   B   has its highest incidence in the 5th decade
   C   is reliably diagnosed by barium swallow
   D   should be assessed endoscopically when surgical resection is
      contemplated

143   Malignant tumours of the oesophagus
   A   are most commonly adenocarcinomas
   B   occur most commonly in males
   C   are most commonly situated in its upper third
   D   commonly spread by lymphatics

140 A **False** the hernial ring is always on the left side of the oesophagus.
    B **True** these are true herniae of the fundus of the stomach into the chest. The cardia remains in its usual abdominal position.
    C **False** there is not usually any incompetence of the cardia so reflux of gastric contents and oesophagitis does not occur.
    D **True** the distension of the intrathoracic portion of the stomach after meals produces a severe 'crushing' pain in the chest and this is often confused with angina.

141 A **True** ulceration of the portion of the stomach inside the hernia is common.
    B **True** bleeding occurs from gastric ulceration or the area of gastritis which is frequently present in the part of the stomach adjacent to the hernial ring.
    C **False** they are rarely seen before middle age and are most common in the elderly. It is generally assumed they are acquired lesions.
    D **False** treatment is usually surgical and is often indicated because of the distressing symptoms, the chronic blood loss and the risk of strangulation or perforation.

142 A **False** the commonest symptom is a progressive unremitting dysphagia.
    B **False** the incidence rises with age and is most common in patients over 70.
    C **True** positive information is yielded by this investigation in more than 95 per cent of patients.
    D **True** this allows biopsy or cytological examination of the lesion by oesophagoscopy. Bronchoscopy should be performed to establish whether the trachea or bronchi are invaded by tumour.

143 A **False** the squamous cell carcinoma is by far the commonest tumour. Adenocarcinomas are almost entirely. confined to the lower end of the oesophagus where they arise from the columnar epithelium adjacent to the cardia.
    B **True** overall, these malignancies are between 2 and 5 times more frequent in males, although cancers of the upper third of the oesophagus occur predominantly in females.
    C **False** about half the malignancies occur in the middle third and about one-third in the lower third.
    D **True** intramural extension, spread to lymph nodes and local spread to invade adjacent structures are all very common. Blood borne metastases are rare.

144   In the treatment of oesophageal cancers
    A surgical excision of the tumour is feasible in the majority of patients
    B radiotherapy is frequently used
    C chemotherapy is of particular value in squamous cell lesions
    D gastrostomy provides good palliation for patients with complete dysphagia

145   Vomiting against a closed glottis
    A may cause a 'spontaneous' rupture of the oesophagus
    B may be followed by severe chest pain and circulatory collapse
    C may cause a laceration of the mucosa of the oesophagogastric junction
    D may cause gastrointestinal bleeding

144 A **False**   the resectability rate is usually less than 30 per cent because of its frequent spread to other mediastinal structures.

B **True**   the squamous cell carcinoma is radiosensitive. Thus, radiotherapy finds a place in palliation of inoperable cases, as an adjunct to surgery pre-and postoperatively and as a sole means of therapy (particularly in upper third cancers).

C **False**   no chemotherapeutic agents have been shown to be useful in the treatment of oesophageal neoplasia.

D **False**   gastrostomy will not relieve this symptom. Complete dysphagia demands early palliation to relieve the distressing symptoms of constantly drooling saliva. Radiotherapy or insertion of a tube through the tumour are more effective.

145 A **True**   there is a rapid increase in intraluminal pressure

B **True**   which may be followed by rupture of the lower end of the oesophagus with expulsion of air and gastric contents into the mediastinum and pleural cavity (usually the left side). This condition is known as the Boerhaave syndrome after the name of the first recorded patient. Immediate surgical repair is required. The mortality is high.

C **True**   this is known as the 'Mallory-Weiss' syndrome. There

D **True**   is no pain associated with the bleeding; barium studies are not as helpful as endoscopy in diagnosis. Surgical measures are occasionally required to stop continuing bleeding.

8 Trachea and thorax

146 The airway of an unconscious patient
A is protected from aspiration of vomit in the semiprone position
B is especially at risk in injuries of the face and neck
C can be effectively protected from vomit by an oropharyngeal tube
D can be effectively protected from aspiration of vomit by a cuffed endotracheal tube

147 The indications for a tracheostomy include
A sputum retention
B an inadequate tidal volume
C a flail chest
D tetanus

148 The complications of a tracheostomy include
A laryngeal stenosis
B erosion of the left brachiocephalic vein
C erosion of the innominate artery
D tracheoesophageal fistula

149 A flail chest wall segment in an injured patient
A demands that frequent blood gas analysis is undertaken
B does not usually require mechanical ventilation
C should be treated by skeletal fixation
D is frequently complicated by myocardial or pulmonary contusion

146 A **True**   in the 'first aid' situation the positioning of the patient
                  head down and semiprone protects him from
                  aspiration.
    B **True**   because of the possibility of direct trauma to the
                  airway.
    C **False**   although this is a simple method of establishing an
                  airway, it does not protect against aspiration.
    D **True**   this is the most effective method of protecting the
                  airway in the unconscious and severely injured
                  patient.

147 A **True**   whenever respiratory function is disturbed by sputum
    B **True**   retention which is resistant to normal
    C **True**   physiotherapeutic manoeuvres, or by an inadequate
    D **True**   tidal volume (because of fatigue or insufficient
                  stability of the chest wall), an elective tracheostomy
                  will allow spontaneous respiration to be more
                  effective by diminishing the dead space and allowing
                  effective bronchial toilet. Assisted respiration will be
                  required in patients with a flail chest (see Q.149) and
                  in those in whom relaxants are being used.

148 A **False**   tracheal stenosis is usually the result of pressure
                  necrosis and inflammation. It can be avoided by
                  careful attention to cuff pressure and the position of
                  the tracheostomy tube.
    B **True**   particularly in children when the vein may be in the
                  root of the neck.
    C **True**   especially in children when a cuffed tube may erode
                  through the thin-walled trachea into the artery.
    D **True**   this is rare, but the likelihood of this complication
                  increases with the time that a cuffed tube is *in situ*.

149 A **True**   respiration is embarrassed by a flail segment and all
    B **False**   except very minor degrees of unstable chest wall
                  require respiratory support with positive pressure
                  ventilation through a cuffed endotracheal tube or
                  tracheostomy. There is thus a need for frequent gas
                  analysis.
    C **False**   surgical attempts to stabilise the chest have generally
                  been superseded by the use of positive pressure
                  ventilation.
    D **True**   myocardial contusion may show ECG changes of a
                  traumatic myocarditis 3 to 4 days post-injury.
                  Pulmonary contusion is demonstrable radiologically
                  after 24 hours.

150   The physical signs associated with crush injuries of the chest include
  A   pulsus paradoxus
  B   subconjunctival haemorrhage
  C   cardiac arrhythmias
  D   surgical emphysema

151   Blunt injuries to the chest
  A   may cause aortic dissection
  B   may produce a flail segment of the chest wall
  C   may, by causing a flail chest wall segment, embarrass expiration
  D   when non-penetrating cannot produce a pneumothorax

152   Open chest wounds
  A   need an immediate thoracotomy
  B   need immediate sealing by any available method
  C   produce mediastinal 'flap'
  D   produce mediastinal shift

153   A pulmonary contusion
  A   is most evident radiologically 1 to 2 days after an injury
  B   does not usually resolve for 3 weeks
  C   does not produce hypoxaemia
  D   may require positive pressure ventilation

150 A **True**   this is most likely after severe crush injuries over the sternum when pericardial or myocardial damage results in haemorrhage into the pericardial cavity and cardiac tamponade.

B **True**   severe crush injuries to the chest cause acute expulsion of blood from the thoracic cavity. Cervicofacial stasis which is recognisable as a swollen blotchy appearance, together with ecchymoses, is then noticed in the upper trunk, head and neck.

C **True**   these are common after any injury affecting mediastinal structures. Atrial fibrillation is probably the commonest.

D **True**   air may leak into the tissues of the mediastinum or chest wall from a damaged lung or bronchus.

151 A **True**   this may be diagnosed by noting unequal pulses in the upper limbs. Occassionally aortic rupture occurs and should be suspected if there is X-ray evidence of widening of the mediastinum. It requires urgent surgery with the use of cardiopulmonary bypass.

B **True**   when several ribs are fractured in two or more places the stability of a segment of the chest wall is impaired.

C **False**   inspiration is hindered because paradoxical movement (inwards on inspiration) of the flail segment prevents the full development of a negative intrathoracic pressure.

D **False**   lacerations of the lungs or bronchi can be produced by sudden deceleration or by rib fractures.

152 A **False**   the first priority is to seal the wound by any method.

B **True**   This is followed by resuscitation and then an exploratory thoracotomy

C **True**   on inspiration there is shift of the mediastinum

D **True**   towards the uninjured side which impairs lung function. On expiration the mediastinum moves back towards the injured side.

153 A **True**   the initial chest X-ray will often not show the extent of the contusion.

B **False**   resolution is complete in about 1 week.

C **False**   larger contusions do embarrass respiratory function

D **True**   and produce hypoxaemia. Mechanical respiratory support is sometimes required.

154 The diagnosis of haemothorax
   A is more easily made on a supine than an erect chest X-ray
   B cannot be made radiologically until more than 400 ml blood
       are present
   C may require needle aspiration of the chest
   D once confirmed means that conservative measures can be
       adhered to

155 A spontaneous pneumothorax
   A is usually the result of pulmonary tuberculosis
   B frequently occurs in patients with pre-existing pulmonary
       disease
   C is usually treated without major surgery
   D usually requires an exploratory thoracotomy

156 In a pleural effusion
   A 500 ml of fluid may not be clinically or radiologically apparent
   B needle biopsy of the pleura provides a diagnosis of the cause
       in more than 90 per cent of cases
   C rapid withdrawal of fluid is advisable in the case of large
       effusions
   D blood staining usually indicates an inflammatory pathology

154 A **False**   the supine film allows the blood to spread more thinly and it is easily missed on this view. Lateral and oblique views are more informative.

     B **True**   even with oblique views quantities smaller than this may be missed.

     C **True**   this should be considered whenever the diagnosis is uncertain.

     D **False**   blood in the pleural cavity usually leads to the development of an organised thrombus and a fibrothorax. Adequate drainage (possibly by thoracotomy) is therefore usually necessary.

155 A **False**   more than 80 per cent occur in non-tuberculous
     B **True**   patients and of these more than half have no obvious pulmonary pathology. Emphysema, bronchitis, bronchiectasis, tuberculosis and neoplasms are the usual causes of the remainder.

     C **True**   most small pneumothoraces may be treated
     D **False**   conservatively. Should the air leak continue to increase or embarrass pulmonary function then water-sealed intercostal catheter drainage may be required for a few days. Thoracotomy is only required for recurrent pneumothoraces and is advised in order to diagnose and repair, by resection or over-sewing the diseased area of lung, or by pleurectomy.

156 A **True**   this quantity of fluid is the minimum necessary to obliterate the costophrenic angles as seen in an erect chest X-ray. Smaller amounts may occasionally be detected radiologically when loculated in an interlobar fissure or between the visceral and parietal pleura.

     B **False**   this diagnostic procedure is only 50 per cent successful. Thus open biopsy of the visceral and parietal walls of the cavity may be necessary.

     C **False**   rapid withdrawal of large amounts of fluid (over 1500 ml) may precipitate acute unilateral pulmonary oedema. Careful clinical and radiological localization of the fluid is necessary. Once the fluid has been located with the exploring needle, this should be carefully maintained in position throughout the procedure.

     D **False**   the commonest cause of a blood stained effusion is an underlying bronchogenic carcinoma.

157   In pulmonary tuberculosis
   A   the primary focus is usually in a lymph node
   B   the primary focus usually heals completely
   C   the lesion is charcterised histologically by the Reed-Sternberg giant cell
   D   fibrosis is rare in the late stages of the disease

158   Bronchial adenomas
   A   are usually carcinoids
   B   are usually cylindromata
   C   are liable to become malignant in 10 per cent of cases
   D   do not usually produce symptoms

159   Adenocarcinoma of the bronchus
   A   is equally common in the two sexes
   B   is closely associated with pipe smoking
   C   has often spread into the pulmonary veins by the time of diagnosis
   D   Accounts for 25 per cent of bronchogenic carcinomas

160   In carcinoma of the broncus
   A   the overall 5-year survival is 25 per cent
   B   the overall 5-year survival is 15 per cent
   C   the mean survival of the inoperable group of patients is 6 to 8 months
   D   the mean survival of the inoperable group of patients is 18 to 24 months

157 A **False**   the primary (Gohn) focus occurs in the periphery of
                   the lung. It is often accompanied by hilar node
                   involvement.
     B **True**   in a few cases, particularly in the first few years of life,
                   widespread blood stream dissemination occurs to
                   produce miliary tuberculosis.
     C **False**   the tubercle consists of an area of central necrosis
                   surrounded by epithelioid cells and multinuclear
                   Langerhan's giant cells.
     D **False**   this is the characteristic finding in the late stages of
                   the disease.

158 A **True**   about 90 per cent are carcinoid and about 8 per cent
                   cylindromata.
     B **False**   the carcinoid tumour may give rise to the carcinoid
                   syndrome if it metastasises to the liver.
     C **True**   but bronchial adenomas are much less common than
                   bronchogenic cancer (ratio 1 : 50).
     D **False**   haemoptysis is the usual presenting complaint but
                   more than half the patients demonstrate
                   bronchiectasis. Occasionally a lung abscess will result
                   from bronchial obstruction.

159 A **False**   it is twice as common in men as in women (squamous
                   and undifferentiated carcinomas are more than 8
                   times commoner in males than in females).
     B **False**   the close relationship of cigarette smoking with
                   squamous and undifferentiated forms of
                   bronchogenic carcinoma is less obvious with
                   adenocarcinoma. There is no certain evidence linking
                   pipe and cigar smoking with lung cancer.
     C **True**   owing to it being found most frequently in the
                   periphery of the lung, it is often diagnosed late when
                   both lymphatic and blood stream spread has taken
                   place.
     D **False**   this cancer accounts for only 10 per cent of all
                   bronchogenic cancers. The majority are divided
                   between the squamous and undifferentiated forms.

160 A **False**   although a 30 per cent 5-year survival rate may be
     B **False**   obtained after complete removal, only 25 per cent of
                   cases are operable and the overall 5-year survival is in
                   the region of 8 per cent
     C **True**   survival in this group is little affected by palliative
     D **False**   surgery, chemotherapy or radiotherapy, although
                   these measures may provide some symptomatic relief.

161 **In the diagnosis of carcinoma of the bronchus**
  A sputum cytology gives 3 per cent false positive results
  B biopsy of an undifferentiated growth is often accompanied by brisk haemorrhage
  C bronchoscopy is diagnostic in 30 to 40 per cent of patients
  D mediastinoscopy permits examination of both sides of the tracheal bifurcation

162 **In Pancoast's syndrome**
  A the right vocal cord is commonly paralysed
  B collateral veins develop over the anterior chest wall
  C nocturnal pain in the upper arm is common
  D the growth is usually an adenocarcinoma of the lung

163 **In carcinoma of the bronchus**
  A the commonest group of symptoms are due to superadded infection
  B the commonest non-metastatic extrapulmonary sign is pulmonary osteodystrophy
  C antidiuretic hormone may be released by the tumour
  D posterior lateral column degeneration is the commonest spinal cord manifestation

161 A **False** false positives are very rare but the diagnostic yield in all but the most experienced laboratories is not high. Therefore, negative results do not exclude cancer.

B **False** the bronchial adenoma is notorious for its vascularity and frequently causes troublesome bleeding after biopsy.

C **True** this investigation allows biopsy of a lesion and the taking of brushings and washings from the bronchial tree. It should preferably be combined with bronchography. It is also very valuable in assessing the operability of the tumour.

D **False** although this investigation is a most useful one in assessing operability of a tumour and the extent of nodal involvement in the mediastinum, the examination is largely limited to the right side, by the presence of the aortic arch on the left.

162 A **False** the syndrome is produced by involvement of the lower part of the brachial plexus and sympathetic chain by an apical lung neoplasm. Typically there is no vagal or recurrent nerve involvement.

B **False** superior vena caval obstruction caused by malignant mediastinal nodes is seen frequently in carcinoma of the bronchus and is not necessarily associated with an apical lung neoplasm or the Pancoast syndrome.

C **True** characteristic of this particular tumour is the development of continuous severe pain over the ulnar apsect of the upper limb, the shoulder and the jaw.

D **False** the commonest tumour is a squamous or an undifferentiated bronchogenic cancer.

163 A **True** these give rise to frequent difficulty in the differential diagnosis, particularly with viral infections which are slow to resolve.

B **True** quite frequently the first sign to appear is the sudden onset of finger clubbing.

C **True** this results in fluid retention and a fall in the serum sodium concentration. Cushing's syndrome is, however, the most common endocrine manifestation of this tumour.

D **True** cerebral and cerebellar degeneration and peripheral neuropathy also occur.

164 Malignant neoplasms of the pleura
  A are usually of epithelial origin
  B may be associated with finger clubbing
  C are the commonest cause of chylothorax
  D can frequently be cured by surgical treatment

165 Pulmonary embolism
  A can be demonstrated at post mortem in 60 per cent of people over the age of 60
  B can usually be diagnosed by a plain chest X-ray
  C of the paradoxical variety has the red and white laminae of originating thrombus in the reverse of the normal order
  D can be effectively treated by infusion of streptokinase through a pulmonary artery catheter

45% on 23/3

164 A **False**   the commonest primary pleural tumours are
mesotheliomata. These are neoplasms of connective
tissue origin and are believed to be related to asbestos
inhalation.

  B **False**   arthralgia, fever and finger clubbing are seen in
association with localised relatively benign
mesotheliomata but not typically with malignant
pleural tumours.

  C **False**   chylothorax is almost always the result of indirect
violence to the chest or surgical trauma. It is
occasionally the result of malignant infiltration of the
thoracic duct.

  D **False**   long term survival of more than 2 years has not been
recorded in any patient with a mesothelioma. Neither
surgery, radiotherapy nor chemotherapy appear to
influence the course of the disease.

165 A **True**   this remarkably high incidence corresponds to the
incidence of clinically silent episodes of lower leg
thrombosis demonstrated in this age group by the I^{125}
labelled fibrinogen technique.

  B **False**   changes are often absent or minimal. A lung scan is
helpful and a pulmonary artery angiogram diagnostic.

  C **False**   a paradoxical embolus is an embolus arising from the
lower limb which enters the systemic circulation
through a patent foramen ovale and produces arterial
occlusion.

  D **True**   this method of local administration of streptokinase
has been effective in producing rapid resolution of the
embolus. It has largely superseded the need to
perform emergency pulmonary embolectomy.

9 Hernia, peritoneum and abdominal trauma

166 The diagnosis of an inguinal hernia
    A in infants often depends on the history given by its mother
    B in the adult is most easily made with the patient in the sitting
        position
    C depends on the hernial sac or cough impulse being felt below
        the inguinal ligament
    D is supported by the presence of a transilluminable scrotal
        swelling

167 Inguinal herniae
    A in children are usually of the indirect type
    B of the indirect type are congenital in origin
    C will regress spontaneously in children
    D in young adults are most commonly of the direct type

168 Strangulated contents of hernial sacs
    A are always accompanied by intestinal obstruction
    B are more common in direct than indirect inguinal herniae
    C are usually irreducible
    D produce local pain and tenderness

169 incisional herniae are related to
    A wound infections
    B anaemia and malnutrition
    C obesity
    D the use of absorbable suture materials

166 A **True**   an inguinal lump may have been noted only when the child is crying, therefore an isolated examination may not reveal it. A slight thickening of the spermatic cord caused by the empty hernial sac may be palpable.

    B **False**   the patient should have his groin inspected and palpated when standing.

    C **False**   inguinal herniae are seen and felt to emerge through the superficial inguinal ring above the inguinal ligament, femoral herniae are found below it.

    D **False**   a hernia is not usually transilluminable (whereas epididymal cysts and hydrocoeles usually are).

167 A **True**   the vast majority of inguinal herniae in childhood are
    B **True**   indirect inguinal herniae within a patent process
    C **False**   vaginalis. They do not obliterate spontaneously and should be treated surgically.

    D **False**   the direct inguinal hernia passes through a diffuse weakness in the transversalis fascia and posterior wall of the inguinal canal. It is thus most common in old age.

168 A **False**   Herniae may produce strangulation of omentum without intestinal involvement. Occasionally only part of the intestinal wall is 'threatened' (a Richter's hernia) and intestinal obstruction may not occur.

    B **False**   direct inguinal herniae are less likely to strangulate for they have a wider neck and a shorter sac.

    C **True**   irreducibility is a sign of incarceration of the hernial
    D **True**   contents and strangulation may be imminent. Strangulation produces pain, local tenderness and, often, discolouration of the overlying tissues.

169 A **True**   these are iatrogenic herniae and the commonest
    B **False**   predisposing cause is an infection of the original
    C **True**   surgical wound. There is a greatly increased incidence
    D **True**   in obese patients, possibly because of the increased incidence of wound haematomata but no definite evidence exists that either anaemia or hypoproteinaemia contributes to their formation. The use of absorbable suture materials to close aponeurotic sheaths is, possibly, a factor in their formation. Catgut loses its tensile strength in 10 to 20 days and aponeuroses do not gain more than 60 per cent of their original strength for 6 to 8 months.

170   Herniae in the umbilical region
A   are always acquired in origin
B   usually occur in males
C   usually require surgical repair in infants
D   rarely strangulate

171   A discharge from the umbilicus
A   may indicate a patent vitello-intestinal duct
B   may indicate an anomaly of the urachus
C   at the time of menstruation may indicate endometriosis
D   in the neonate is of no immediate clinical significance

172   An exomphalos
A   is a congenital defect of the urethra
B   is a congenital defect of the anterior abdominal wall
C   is otherwise known as gastroschisis
D   needs urgent surgical treatment

170 A **False**   they are of two types: the infantile type which
                      presents at birth is due to a congenital weakness in
                      the umbilicus, and the acquired adult type which most
                      frequently occurs in obese elderly patients is due to a
                      weakness occurring in the linea alba just above the
                      umbilicus. This latter type is known as a
                      para-umbilical hernia.
     B **False**   there is not an increased incidence in males.
     C **False**   those of the infantile type frequently close
                      spontaneously before the age of 2 years, especially if
                      the defect is less than 1 cm in diameter.
     D **False**   the para-umbilical hernia is particularly prone to
                      strangulation, and surgical repair is thus usually
                      indicated in this group.

171 A **True**   when the vitello-intestinal duct fails to disappear and
                      remains patent throughout its length, a congenital
                      small bowel fistula exists. Other related anomalies
                      include Meckel's diverticulum and a fibrous
                      congenital vitello-intestinal band.
     B **True**   a patent urachus results in the intermittent discharge
                      of urine from the umbilicus.
     C **True**   this is rare; the discharge is bloody and arises from
                      ectopic endometrial tissue.
     D **False**   in addition to the congenital defects already referred
                      to, infection of the umbilicus (omphalitis) in the new
                      born is potentially dangerous because of its rapid
                      spread to the surrounding abdominal wall,
                      peritoneum and, via incompletely obliterated
                      umbilical vessels, to the liver.

172 A **False**   exomphalos is a herniation of intra-abdominal viscera
     B **True**   through the umbilical ring. It is covered by a
     C **False**   peritoneal sac which often ruptures after birth.
     D **True**   Gastroschisis is a congenital defect of the abdominal
                      wall and has no membranous covering. A proportion
                      of the less severe cases can be treated by primary
                      closure but the majority with an intact sac are treated
                      by dressing with 2 per cent mercurochrome. This
                      allows epithelisation to occur and the ventral hernia
                      can be treated at a later date. A ruptured exomphalos
                      or gastroschisis needs urgent closure. In the larger
                      defects this may be achieved by covering with silastic
                      sheeting which allows epithelisation and staged
                      closure to be undertaken.

173   **Widespread carcinomatous involvement of the peritoneum**
  A   is frequently confirmed by abdominal paracentesis
  B   can often be diagnosed by rectal examination
  C   indicates that the primary neoplasm is abdominal in origin
  D   is usually associated with jaundice

174   **Blunt injuries to the abdomen**
  A   may cause peritonitis
  B   may cause intestinal obstruction
  C   may cause acute gastroduodenal ulceration
  D   rarely need urgent laparotomy

175   **Car seat belts (lap diagonal) when properly adjusted**
  A   prevent injuries to the abdominal viscera
  B   may cause small bowel injuries
  C   do not reduce the incidence of head injuries amongst car
      passengers involved in a road traffic accident
  D   protect the cervical spine during sudden acceleration

176   **Indication of a serious intra-abdominal injury in a comatose patient may be gained by**
  A   abdominal paracentesis
  B   the observation of pattern bruising on the abdominal wall
  C   falling haemoglobin values
  D   the presence of diarrhoea

173 A **True**   cytological examination of a sample of ascitic fluid often reveals the presence of exfoliated neoplastic cells.

   B **True**   the rectovesical or recto-uterine pouch is frequently the site of peritoneal metastatic deposits.

   C **False**   disseminated breast cancer frequently results in peritoneal deposits and ascites.

   D **False**   although metastases in the liver and porta hepatis are frequently present, there is no close association between peritoneal deposits and jaundice.

174 A **True**   crushing or tearing of the bowel may occur and result in a perforation.

   B **True**   bleeding from a submucosal vessel may produce an intramural haematoma large enough to cause intestinal obstruction.

   C **True**   'stress' ulcers of the stomach and duodenum may follow any hypotensive episode.

   D **False**   the signs of peritonitis, or of intra-abdominal haemorrhage necessitate urgent laparotomy.

175 A **False**   serious injuries to bowel, mesenteric vessels,
   B **True**   pancreas and kidney may still occur during sudden deceleration. It should be emphasised that the injuries would probably have been more serious had a belt not been worn.

   C **False**   seat belts largely prevent dashboard and windscreen head injuries occuring.

   D **False**   'whiplash' injuries to the cervical spine can occur during a sudden acceleration even when seat belts are worn. They may be reduced by the introduction of head rests.

176 A **True**   aspiration of blood or purulent peritoneal fluid suggests visceral injury.

   B **True**   when the pattern of clothing is imprinted on the abdominal wall, it implies that a severe crush injury has occured.

   C **True**   this may denote a splenic or liver rupture.
   D **False**

177 Penetrating wounds of the abdomen
    A can be adequately explored by a probe
    B frequently result in acquired abdominal wall herniae
    C may be managed by careful observation, laparotomy being indicated if signs of peritonitis occur
    D can be treated conservatively if the weapon is less than 3 cm long

178 Urinary tract injuries
    A are usually accompanied by some degree of haematuria
    B require an urgent intravenous pyelogram and possibly a cystogram
    C involving the kidney require urgent surgery
    D which demonstrate urine extravasating from the bladder are generally managed conservatively

179 Injuries to the urethra
    A are usually confined to the male
    B are often caused by road traffic accidents
    C are readily diagnosed on intravenous pyelography
    D require urgent surgical treatment

180 Patients with renal trauma
    A usually present with haematuria
    B usually require surgical management
    C always require an intravenous pyelogram
    D often present with acute renal failure

177 A **False**   the shuttering and overriding actions of the
                  abdominal wall muscles prevent full exploration with
                  a probe.
    B **False**   this is no more common than after laparotomy.
    C **True**   if the patient is observed carefully, an experienced
                  clinician may avoid an unnecessary laparotomy.
    D **False**   compression of the abdomen wall occurs during
                  penetration, thus allowing short objects to enter the
                  peritoneal cavity and the viscera.

178 A **True**   the amount of haematuria does not relate to the
                 degree of damage to the urinary tract.
    B **True**   these two investigations will, in most cases, localise
                 the injury, establish whether the patient has two
                 kidneys and determine the function of each.
    C **False** the early management of the injured kidney is, in most
                 cases, by observation.
    D **False** urgent surgery is indicated once this diagnosis is
                 made.

179 A **False** fractures of the pelvis in either sex may result in a torn
    B **True**   membranous urethra. In the male the prostate and
                 bladder may then be displaced upwards.
    C **False** failure to pass urine, after a pelvic injury, should
                 arouse suspicion and if gentle catheterisation is not
                 possible then urethrograms or laparotomy will be
                 required to establish the diagnosis.
    D **True**   diversion of the urinary stream and restoration of
                 urethral continuity should be undertaken in every case
                 in order to avoid extravasation, periurethral fibrosis
                 and stricture formation.

180 A **True**   the commonest results of blunt trauma to the kidney
    B **False** are relatively minor contusions or lacerations to the
                 renal parenchyma. These cause loin pain and overt or
                 microscopic haematuria. Surgery is not necessary
                 except in the rare cases of major lacerations or
                 injuries to the renal pedicle.
    C **True**   this is a most important investigation. Not only may it
                 confirm the suspected injury but it will also present
                 evidence of the presence or absence of the
                 contralateral kidney.
    D **False** this is rare but may follow severe injury to a solitary
                 kidney or bilateral severe injuries.

181 **The spleen**
   A is the commonest organ injured in blunt abdominal trauma
   B usually continues to bleed once its capsule is torn and its pulp
      lacerated
   C either bleeds immediately or not at all after a pulp injury
   D should be removed if there has been a laceration of its
      capsule

182 **Traumatic rupture of the spleen**
   A not infrequently presents more than 7 days after the causative
      injury
   B frequently presents with shoulder tip pain
   C may be diagnosed by paracentesis
   D may, in the absence of hypovolaemia, be treated
      conservatively   40% on 24/3

181 A **True**   on account of its thin capsule, proximity to the ribs
             and its relatively mobile nature.
      B **True**   a torn capsule with a pulp laceration is unlikely to stop
      C **False**   bleeding. A pulp laceration lying deep to an intact
      D **True**   capsule may produce a sub capsular haematoma
             which develops over a period of days, weeks or
             months. Delayed spontaneous haemorrhage will
             almost certainly ensue. It is advisable to remove any
             spleen which has any signs of trauma.

182 A **True**   in 20 per cent of cases the rupture is delayed for up to
             2 weeks after the injury. This is usually due to a
             delayed rupture of a subcapsular haematoma into the
             peritoneal cavity.
      B **True**   this is usually left sided and indicates the left sided
             diaphragmatic irritation that is common in this
             condition.
      C **True**   a four quadrant paracentesis through a fine needle is
             valuable in the investigation of any suspected
             abdominal injury. A negative paracentesis does not
             exclude the possibility of a haemoperitoneum but a
             positive aspirate will encourage early laparotomy.
      D **False**   any suspicion of a ruptured spleen indicates the need
             for laparotomy. Delayed haemorrhage, when it
             occurs, is frequently catastrophic.

10 The acute abdomen

183 Acute abdominal pain which is
A colicky in nature indicates obstruction of a hollow viscus
B continuous is typical of inflammation
C maximal in the right loin is typical of duodenal ulceration
D in the right upper quadrant accentuated by inspiration is typical of cholecystitis

184 In the acute abdomen, vomiting
A occurring soon after the onset of colicky pain often indicates pathology outside the gastrointestinal tract
B of fluid containing no bile is characteristic of small bowel obstruction
C of faeculent fluid usually indicates a gastro-colic fistula
D is a common early accompaniment of gastroduodenal perforation

185 Faeculent vomiting
A is commonly seen after upper gastrointestinal tract bleeding
B indicates large bowel obstruction
C indicates bacterial proliferation in the upper intestinal tract
D suggests a gastro-colic fistula

186 A patient with generalised peritonitis
A usually has an elevated temperature and pulse rate
B characteristically complains of spasmodic severe pain which causes him to be restless
C characteristically vomits
D will usually have a rapid and deep respiratory pattern

183 A **True**   ureteric colic arises in the lumbar region and spreads
                    down via the iliac fossa towards the external genitalia;
                    biliary colic will characteristically be maximal in the
                    right upper quadrant; intestinal colic will be referred
                    to the midline anteriorly.

     B **True**   whether this arises from infection, haemorrhage or
                    ischaemia.

     C **False**   duodenal pain is felt in the epigastrium. Loin pain is
                    usually of renal origin.

     D **True**   be aware that diaphragmatic irritation from pleural or
                    pulmonary pathology may produce the same kind of
                    pain.

184 A **True**   both biliary and renal colic produce 'reflex' vomiting
                    coincident with the pain. This will, however, also
                    occur with a high small bowel obstruction.

     B **False**   this almost always indicates gastric pathology,
                    particularly pyloric stenosis

     C **False**   this is a very rare cause of faeculent vomiting. The
                    usual cause is well developed lower small bowel
                    obstruction. Bacterial proliferation and decomposition
                    of the stagnant bowel contents causes this faeculent
                    change.

     D **False**   vomiting is an uncommon early symptom in this
                    condition.

185 A **False**   small bowel obstruction always results in bacterial
     B **False**   proliferation and decomposition of the small bowel
     C **True**   contents then occurs. The smell and appearance of
                    such vomitus is faeculent. Altered blood is usually
                    darker and less foul smelling. Faeculent vomiting is a
                    late (and relatively infrequent) sign of large bowel
                    obstruction.

     D **False**   in this rare condition, if vomiting occurs then the
                    vomitus may contain faeces. It does not have the
                    homogeneity of faeculent vomiting.

186 A **True**   though these may take a few hours to develop.
     B **False**   the pain is severe, constant and widespread and the
                    patient lies motionless since movement exacerbates
                    the pain.

     C **True**   this is almost constantly present. At first it is reflex in
                    nature and the volume is small but as the effects of the
                    ensuing paralytic ileus develop the vomit increases in
                    volume.

     D **False**   the respiratory movements though rapid are shallow
                    for diaphragmatic and abdominal wall movements
                    increase the pain.

187   Perforated duodenal ulcers

   A occur most frequently in men

   B are usually preceded by an exacerbation of ulcer symptoms

   C are usually accompanied by a leucocytosis

   D produce abdominal tenderness which is most marked in the epigastrium

188   A perforated duodenal ulcer

   A usually lies on the anterior or superior surface of the duodenum

   B usually presents with the acute onset of severe back pain

   C produces radiological evidence of free gas in the peritoneum in over 90 per cent of the patients

   D is usually treated by simple closure of the perforation

189   Congenital pyloric stenosis

   A occurs more commonly in male children

   B usually presents in the first few days of life

   C presents with bile-stained vomiting

   D is usually diagnosed on clinical examination

187 A **True**   it is 3 to 4 times more common in males.
     B **True**   the majority of patients have had a recent worsening
                    of ulcer symptoms. A small minority have no previous
                    dyspeptic history.
     C **True**   the leucocyte count usually rises within a few hours
                    due to developing peritonitis.
     D **True**   as in all cases of generalised peritonitis, the
                    abdominal tenderness and rigidity are most marked
                    over the causative lesion.

188 A **True**   penetrating posterior ulcers usually bleed after
                    erosion of the gastroduodenal artery; anterior ulcers
                    perforate rather than bleed.
     B **False**   by far the commonest presentation is the acute onset
                    of severe epigastric pain which rapidly spreads to the
                    whole abdomen.
     C **False**   less than 75 per cent of perforated ulcers show free
                    gas under the diaphragm on an erect film of the
                    abdomen.
     D **True**   for acute ulcers and small chronic ulcers this is
                    advised. In perforation of large ulcers definitive
                    surgery, i.e. vagotomy and pyloroplasty or partial
                    gastrectomy is usually preferred providing that
                    peritoneal contimination is neither extensive nor well
                    established.

189 A **True**   boys are affected four times as commonly as girls.
                    There is some evidence of a hereditary tendency.
     B **False**   the signs of pyloric obstruction usually present after
                    the second week of life. By this time oedema of the
                    pyloric mucosa contributes to the narrowing
                    produced by the hypertrophied pyloric muscle to
                    cause obstruction.
     C **False**   projectile vomiting, particularly after feeds, occurs,
                    but this is not bilestained since the obstruction is
                    proximal to the ampulla of Vater.
     D **True**   if the abdomen is examined after the infant has been
                    fed, forceful transverse peristaltic waves can usually
                    be seen passing from left to right across the upper
                    abdomen and the abnormal mass of hypertrophied
                    muscle, the 'pyloric tumour', becomes palpable.
                    Surgical treatment is indicated once fluid and
                    electrolyte imbalance has been corrected.

190   Acute appendicitis
   A   is most common in the 30 to 40 year age group
   B   characteristically presents with a high temperature
   C   is often associated with painful extension of the right hip
   D   may produce haematuria and pyuria

191   Appendicitis is
   A   more common in females
   B   distributed evenly throughout the world's population
   C   more likely to occur if the appendix is in the retrocaecal
        position
   D   commonly the result of appendicular obstruction

192   The physical signs of early appendicitis
   A   are generally of more diagnostic value than the patient's
        history
   B   usually include muscle guarding in the right iliac fossa
   C   usually include a pyrexia above 38.5°C
   D   do not include rectal tenderness

193   Patients with early appendicitis
   A   usually present with central abdominal pain
   B   rarely present with anorexia
   C   have usually vomited on one or two occasions
   D   usually complain of similar attacks of pain in the previous few
        weeks

190 A **False**   the peak incidence is in the 15 to 25 year age group. It
                     is uncommon in the very young and the very old (but
                     more dangerous and difficult to diagnose).
     B **False**   temperature and pulse are frequently normal early in
                     the disease. The temperature rarely exceeds 38°C
                     unless perforation or abscess formation has occurred.
     C **True**   the retrocaecal position is the most common and in
                     this position the inflamed appendix may produce
                     spasm of iliopsoas and painful limited extension of
                     the right hip. This is a useful diagnostic sign.
     D **True**   right sided renal and ureteric colic are frequently
                     confused with appendicitis. The detection of red cells
                     in the urine usually indicates urinary calculi as the
                     cause. However an inflamed appendix that lies
                     adjacent to the right ureter or bladder may produce
                     urinary symptoms such as haematuria and pyuria.

191 A **False**   the incidence is the same in both sexes.
     B False   the disease is uncommon in the underdeveloped
                     countries of the Third World.
     C **False**   though this is the commonest position of the
                     appendix, it carries no increased risk of appendicitis.
     D **True**   appendicitis follows obstruction of the appendicular
                     lumen due either to lymphoid hyperplasia (which is
                     particularly common in children), a faecolith (which is
                     found in almost half the cases) or, rarely, to a tumour
                     or stricture.

192 A **False**   usually the reverse is true.
     B **True**   this resistance to palpation is a guide to the severity of
                     the inflammation and it progresses to involuntary
                     rigidity.
     C **False**   a milder pyrexia is common. High fever is uncommon
                     until perforation or abscess formation occurs.
     D **False**   a rectal examination should always be performed.
                     Rectal tenderness in the pouch of Douglas may
                     provide the only positive evidence of appendicitis
                     when the inflamed organ lies in the pelvis.

193 A **True**   this is felt most severely in the umbilical region. In a
                     few cases such a history is not obtained.
     B **False**   anorexia is almost always noted in patients with
                     appendicitis.
     C **True**   this follows the abdominal pain and may be reflex in
                     nature.
     D **False**   though recurrent appendicitis occasionally occurs it is
                     rare. A history of previous abdominal pain should
                     alert the clinician to think of other causes of the
                     abdominal pain.

194   Investigation of a case of acute appendicitis
    A   will usually reveal a polymorphonuclear leucocytosis
    B   often shows microscopic haematuria
    C   usually reveals haemoconcentration
    D   often reveals fluid levels in the right iliac fossa on an erect
         X-ray of the abdomen

**195   Likely differential diagnoses in a young woman with
        appendicitis include**
    A   ovulatory pain
    B   ruptured ectopic pregnancy
    C   colonic diverticulitis
    D   caecal carcinoma

196   Appendicectomy should be undertaken
    A   after laparotomy reveals a diagnosis of mesenteric adenitis
    B   immediately in adult patients with an appendix abscess
    C   in patients with a gangrenous appendix
    D   in patients with chronic appendicitis

197   Obstruction of the lumen of the appendix may lead to
    A   mucosal ulceration
    B   gangrenous appendicitis
    C   a perforated appendix
    D   intussusception of the appendix

**198   In the differential diagnosis of appendicitis in an infant it is
        important to consider**
    A   ileo-ileal intussusception
    B   basal pneumonia
    C   Henoch-Schoenlein purpura
    D   torsion of an ovarian cyst

194 A **True**   too much emphasis should not be placed on
    B **True**   laboratory tests for their discriminatory value is slight.
    C **False**   Though there is usually a leucocytosis this is not
                   constant. About one-quarter of patients will show
                   leucocytes or red cells in the urine but there is rarely a
                   raised haematocrit in the early case.
    D **False**   abdominal radiology is not often helpful. When there
                   is radiological evidence of appendicitis (such as the
                   absence of small bowel gas in the right iliac fossa, gas
                   under the diaphragm or a scoliosis concave to the
                   right)), the diagnosis is usually clinically obvious.

195 A **True**   midcycle ovulatory pain lasts for only a few hours
    B **True**   often there is a history of a missed menstruation and
                   the presence of a tender tubal mass is noted on pelvic
                   examination.
    C **False**   colonic diverticulitis and caecal cancer may mimic
    D **False**   appendicitis, but it is extremely uncommon for these
                   to occur in this age group

196 A **True**   the procedure is prophylactic and carries little
                   additional morbidity and mortality.
    B **False**   it is usually wisest to surgically drain the abscess and
                   unless the appendix can be removed easily it should
                   be left for an interval appendicectomy some 2 months
                   later.
    C **True**   in all cases.
    D **True**   this disputed condition occurs but is not common.

197 A **True**   luminal obstruction leads to oedema and distension
    B **True**   of the distal appendix, mucosal ulcers appear and as
    C **True**   the distension increases the venous drainage and
                   arterial supply are impeded and gangrenous
                   perforation may occur. Peritonitis may then follow
                   and the mortality rises.
    D **False**   this is not related.

198 A **True**   screaming and intermittent abdominal colic, a short
                   history of melaena and palpation of a sausage-shaped
                   mass may indicate an intussusception.
    B **True**   diaphragmatic pleurisy may produce referred pain in
                   the lower abdomen.
    C **True**   a haematoma of the small bowel wall may mimic
                   appendicitis but the presence of a purpuric rash and
                   joint pains should arouse suspicion of
                   Henoch-Schoenlein purpura.
    D **False**   this is very uncommon before puberty.

199   Acute non-specific mesenteric lymphadenitis
   A   is commonest between 5 and 12 years of age
   B   is usually associated with an upper respiratory tract infection
   C   is usually associated with cervical lymphadenopathy
   D   is characterised by enlarged mesenteric lymph nodes which
        are infected by gram-negative organisms

**200   Abdominal distension in mechanical intestinal obstruction is
         produced in part by**
   A   swallowed air
   B   carbon dioxide produced in the bowel
   C   increased intestinal secretions proximal to the obstruction
   D   decreased intestinal absorption proximal to the obstruction

201   The level of intestinal obstruction can be determined by
   A   questioning the patient
   B   examining the patient
   C   radiological examination of the patient
   D   repeated measurements of the patient's girth

199 A **True**   although it is less common than appendicitis in this age group.

B **True**   this is commonly coexistent with, or precedes the vague, colicky, lower abdominal pain by a few days.

C **True**   there is frequently pharyngeal injection. Examination of the abdomen reveals tenderness which is higher, more medial and more variable in position than appendicitis. The leucocyte count is moderately raised to 12 000 to 15 000/mm^3.(12 000 to 15 000/μl).

D **False**   although mesenteric lymph node enlargement is characteristically present, cultures of the nodes are usually sterile.

200 A **True**   nitrogen is not readily absorbed by the intestine, thus more than 70 per cent of the accumulated gas comes from swallowed air.

B **False**   though large quantities of carbon dioxide are produced in the bowel, accumulation does not occur because this gas is readily absorbed.

C **True**   in the distended bowel there is a gross disturbance of
D **True**   the usual absorption/secretion activities of the intestinal mucosa. Both increased secretion and decreased absorption of fluid have been shown to occur in a distended bowel proximal to an obstruction.

201 A **True**   in high small bowel obstruction vomiting occurs soon after the onset of pain whereas in large bowel obstruction vomiting appears much later if at all. Small bowel colic is felt in the central abdomen; large bowel colic in the suprapubic region. Constipation is an early symptom in large bowel obstruction.

B **True**   in large bowel obstruction distension is greater and tends to be most marked in the flanks. The distension of small bowel obstruction is central abdominal.

C **True**   in small bowel obstruction there is very little gas in the colon. Colonic distension can usually be distinguished from small bowel distension by haustral markings which occupy only part of the transverse diameter of the bowel. In distended small bowel, mucosal folds, the valvulae conniventes, can be seen traversing the whole diameter.

D **False**   except in high small bowel obstruction progressive increase in the patient's abdominal girth is a feature of all types of intestinal obstruction.

202 **Acute small bowel obstruction**
  A is commonly caused by postoperative adhesions
  B accompanied by the signs of peritonitis, suggests bowel strangulation
  C is often associated with a raised serum amylase
  D generally produces abdominal distension within 2 to 3 hours of onset

203 **In the treatment of intestinal obstruction**
  A nasogastric suction should be instituted preoperatively
  B intravenous fluid replacement is essential
  C immediate surgery is essential
  D surgery should be restricted to those cases where strangulation is diagnosed

204 **Emergency treatment of a mechanical obstruction of the large bowel may include**
  A enemata
  B exteriorisation and resection of the lesion
  C a transverse colostomy
  D an ileo-transverse colostomy

202 A **True**   adhesions and external herniae are the two
                  commonest causes. A careful inspection for surgical
                  scars and of the hernial orifices must therefore be
                  routine.
      B **True**   a rising temperature and pulse rate and local
                  abdominal tenderness and rigidity, all indicate that
                  strangulation is developing. Operative treatment is
                  then an urgent necessity.
      C **True**   the serum amylase is frequently raised to twice
                  normal values but should not be confused with the
                  very high values usually seen in the initial stages of
                  acute pancreatitis.
      D **False**   central abdominal distension usually appears after 12
                  to 24 hours and may be absent in high small bowel
                  obstruction.

203 A **True**   aspiration via a nasogastric tube, though having little
      B **True**   effect on the distended bowel, minimises further
                  distension by removing swallowed air. It also reduces
                  the risk of aspiration of vomit. All patients with
                  intestinal obstruction will have abnormal fluid and
                  electrolyte losses — these must be made good by the
                  intravenous administration of isotonic saline, often
                  with potassium supplements.
      C **False**   although in many cases the most appropriate
                  treatment is surgical relief of the obstruction, this
                  should not be performed until careful attention has
                  been paid to correcting fluid and electrolyte
                  deficiencies and nasogastric suction has been
                  instituted
      D **False**   strangulation is a serious complication adding
                  peritonitis to the pathophysiology of intestinal
                  obstruction. This is reflected in a high mortality rate of
                  more than 25 per cent, and therefore surgery is
                  preferable before this complication develops.

204 A **True**   faecal impaction is a cause of large bowel obstruction
                  in the elderly. It may be effectively treated by enemata
                  though disimpaction under general anaesthetic is
                  frequently necessary.
      B **True**   each of these procedures may have some part to play.
                  It is usually unsafe
      C **True**   to attempt resection of the obstructing lesion with
                  primary anastomosis.
      D **True**   and the majority of cases are managed in the first
                  instance by these simpler methods which permit safe
                  decompression of the proximal bowel.

205   Strangulation of the bowel
    A   commonly complicates closed loop obstruction
    B   is difficult to distinguish from simple intestinal obstruction
    C   is accompanied by bleeding into the affected bowel
    D   frequently causes peritonitis

206   Small bowel obstruction often results in
    A   hyperkalaemia
    B   metabolic alkalosis
    C   oliguria
    D   hypovolaemia

207   Large bowel obstruction
    A   is most commonly caused by diverticular disease of the colon
    B   has its maximum incidence before the age of 50
    C   frequently presents with nausea and vomiting
    D   usually heralds its onset with constant suprapubic pain

205 A **True**   when the bowel lumen is closed at two points along
                 its length the raised intraluminal pressure results in
                 impairment of the blood supply to the affected loop
                 and strangulation frequently occurs.
    B **False** strangulation should be suspected in any patient with
                 intestinal obstruction who demonstrates signs of local
                 or generalised peritonitis.
    C **True**   blood and plasma are lost from the strangulated
                 portion and trapped in it following venous obstruction
                 and capillary leakage. As an approximate guide, one
                 litre of blood may be lost per metre of strangulated
                 bowel.
    D **True**   the ischaemic segment of bowel is permeable to the
                 increased numbers of bacteria and their toxins. This
                 toxic fluid produces peritonitis and its absorption into
                 the general circulation can cause cardiovascular
                 collapse.

206 A **False** potassium is lost in intestinal secretions, in vomiting
    B **True**   and in abnormal renal losses which follow attempts to
    C **True**   conserve hydrogen ions in the metabolic alkalosis that
    D **True**   accompanies proximal small bowel obstruction
                 dehydration rapidly develops due to loss of fluid into
                 the distended bowel, diminished fluid intake and
                 vomiting. Haemoconcentration, hypovolaemia and
                 oliguria thus rapidly appear.

207 A **False** colonic cancer is the most common cause, followed
                 by diverticular disease and sigmoid volvulus. Most of
                 the obstructing cancers are in the descending and
                 sigmoid colon.
    B **False** this is a disease of the elderly.
    C **False** these symptoms are usually absent until the late
                 stages of the disease, particularly when the ileocaecal
                 valve is competent.
    D **False** the visceral pain produced is vague but colicky and
                 felt in the lower abdomen.

208   Patients with acute colonic diverticulitis
   A   often given a history of recent lower abdominal colic
   B   often present with a pyrexia
   C   can be frequently diagnosed on sigmoidoscopic appearances
   D   frequently develop faecal peritonitis

209   Acute volvulus of the colon
   A   occurs most commonly in the transverse colon
   B   produces severe abdominal distension
   C   produces characteristic radiological appearances
   D   may be successfully treated without surgery

210   Acute pancreatitis typically
   A   is accompanied by hypercalcaemia
   B   produces paralytic ileus
   C   is associated with a pleural effusion
   D   produces pyloric stenosis

208 A **True**   these symptoms of diverticular disease frequently
               precede the acute attack.

   B **True**   temperatures of 38°C and above may indicate the
               presence of a pericolic abscess.

   C **False**   though oedema of the rectosigmoid junction may
               occasionally be seen, the more inaccessible pelvic
               colon is the site of the pathology, and out of reach of
               the sigmoidoscope.

   D **False**   rupture of a pericolic abscess may lead to generalised
               peritonitis. This complication, which carries a high
               mortality, is rare. The inflammation more frequently
               localises as a pericolic abscess.

209 A **False**   the commonest site of colonic volvulus is the sigmoid
               colon. Caecal volvulus occurs less frequently. The
               transverse colon rarely undergoes volvulus.

   B **True**   abdominal distension is usually severe. Sigmoid
               volvulus often produces distension which is maximal
               on the right side.

   C **True**   gross colonic distension is always present; sigmoid
               volvulus characteristically produces two obvious fluid
               levels which may be at different levels. A barium
               enema will reveal, at the lowest point of torsion a
               typical 'corkscrew' or 'Birds beak' constriction.

   D **False**   *True*   strangulation frequently results *but may 1° be treated c*
               flatus tube

210 A **False**   hypocalcaemia is a frequent complication occuring
               within a few days of the onset. Though it is frequently
               stated to be a consequence of saponification of
               retroperitoneal fat, this is almost certainly a too facile
               explanation and the true cause is still unknown.

   B **True**   even mild attacks generally produce a segmental ileus
               of the overlying jejunal loops. The distended bowel in
               the upper abdomen produces characteristic
               radiological appearances.

   C **True**   most commonly a left sided effusion, due to
               subdiaphragmatic inflammation.

   D **False**   however there is frequently distortion of the duodenal
               loop on a barium meal.

211   Acute pancreatitis
   A   often simulates a perforated peptic ulcer in its presentation
   B   often presents with the signs of hypovolaemia
   C   can readily be distinguished from other causes of acute
       abdominal pain by the presence of a raised serum amylase
   D   frequently has a raised concentration of urinary amylase

212   The treatment of acute pancreatitis
   A   is largely nonspecific and supportive
   B   should include a laparotomy in the majority of cases
   C   should routinely include the administration of calcium
   D   should routinely include the administration of antibiotics

213   Childhood intussusception
   A   usually presents during the first year of life
   B   is frequently ileocolic
   C   can usually be diagnosed without X-ray examination of the
       abdomen
   D   rarely requires surgical treatment

211 A **True**   the disease varies in severity and the epigastric pain
                     may be as severe as that of a perforated peptic ulcer. It
                     commonly radiates to the back and then must be
                     distinguished from a ruptured or dissecting aortic
                     aneurysm.
     B **True**   in a severe attack there is considerable retroperitoneal
                     inflammation and sequestration of fluid which results
                     in hypovolaemia and shock.
     C **False**   although in most cases the serum amylase rises
     D **True**   within 8 hours of the onset and remains elevated for 2
                     to 3 days only a rise of approximately four times the
                     normal value will certainly distinguish pancreatitis
                     from the other causes of hyperamylasaemia, viz.
                     gallstones, perforated peptic ulcer, small bowel
                     obstruction and mesenteric thrombosis. There is a
                     more constant rise in urinary amylase values in
                     pancreatitis than in the above conditions.

212 A **True**   hypovolaemia should be corrected, continuous
                     nasogastric suction will relieve distension and reduce
                     pancreatic secretion while pain relief can usually be
                     achieved with pethidine
     B **False**   most cases will improve on the above therapy but
                     laparotomy is advised if the patient is deteriorating or
                     if a fever or abdominal mass appears. Usually
                     removal of the necrotic tissue and drainage of the area
                     is all that can be undertaken.
     C **False**   it should only be given in those patients who have
                     clinical or biochemical evidence of hypocalcaemia.
     D **False**   antibiotics are essential in the treatment of any
                     infective complications but their prophylactic use is
                     debatable.

213 A **True**   the average age of presentation is gradually
     B **True**   becoming younger. The cause is obscure. It is
                     suggested lymphatic hyperplasia secondary to virus
                     infections or a change in the infant's diet on weaning,
                     may produce a submucosal swelling in the intestinal
                     wall which initiates the intussusception.
     C **True**   sudden colicky pain, often with the passage of bloody
                     stools, suggests the diagnosis — the palpation of a
                     sausage-shaped mass in the right upper quadrant is
                     confirmatory.
     D **False**   providing no signs of intestinal strangulation exist
                     then *gentle* reduction by means of a barium enema
                     may be attempted under fluoroscopic control. The
                     majority of patients, however, require surgical
                     intervention.

214   Meconium ileus
A   is the presenting feature in the majority of patients with cystic fibrosis
B   is associated with achlorhydria
C   presents with a distended abdomen and bilious vomiting
D   may be effectively treated with acetylcysteine

215   Neonatal duodenal obstruction
A   may be associated with Down's syndrome
B   is more frequently found in premature infants
C   typically presents with gross abdominal distension
D   usually presents with vomiting of bile stained fluid

216   Acute gastric dilatations
A   may follow spinal injuries
B   may cause dehydration and hypovolaemia
C   may cause haemorrhagic ulceration
D   requires urgent surgical treatment

217   Acute superior mesenteric artery occlusion
A   characteristically presents with sudden pain and tenderness of increasing intensity
B   is frequently accompanied by overt or occult blood loss in the stools
C   frequently produces peritonitis
D   can usually be diagnosed on plain abdominal X-rays

214 A **False**   only about 10 per cent of patients with cystic fibrosis have meconium ileus.

B **False**   no abnormalities of gastric secretion occur in this syndrome. There is an associated deficiency of pancreatic function.

C **True**   distal ileal obstruction occurs due to abnormally viscous meconium.

D **True**   this obstruction must usually be relieved surgically or, in mild cases, by the detergent action of orally administered acetylcystcine or gastrografin, a hypertonic contrast medium.

215 A **True**   more than 20 per cent of such infants will also have Down's syndrome.

B **False**   there is not an increased frequency in premature infants.

C **False**   the obstruction is high and so abdominal distension is usually absent.

D **True**   vomiting is frequent, and usually contains bile since the obstruction is usually distal to the ampulla of Vater.

216 A **True**   though the mechanism is not known; the commonest cause is Britain is due to inadequate nasogastric drainage after abdominal surgery.

B **True**   there is gastric hypersecretion. Vomiting and diminished fluid intake produce dehydration and hypovolaemia frequently follows.

C **True**   the vomitus may be blood stained. Untreated cases have been followed by spontaneous rupture of the stomach.

D **True**   effective nasogastric suction is all that is required. All attempts at surgical drainage have been disastrous.

217 A **True**   the pain is often more severe than the abdominal tenderness suggests.

B **True**   intestinal blood loss is almost invariably present and results from haemorrhagic infarction of the bowel mucosa.

C **True**   ischaemia of the bowel leads to the bacteria of the bowel 'leaking' into the peritoneal cavity with catastrophic results.

D **False**   X-rays are usually unhelpful. Occasionally intra-hepatic gas is seen as the ominous result of gas forming organisms ascending via the portal vein to the liver.

218   A ruptured ectopic pregnancy
   A usually occurs in the first month of pregnancy
   B usually presents with severe lower abdominal pain
   C frequently presents with hypovolaemic shock
   D can usually be diagnosed by pelvic examination

219   Acute salpingitis
   A usually occurs in the first month of pregnancy
   B is frequently associated with vomiting
   C often presents with vaginal discharge
   D presents with uterine tenderness

220   A ruptured ovarian cyst
   A most frequently occur premenstrually
   B may cause peritonitis
   C most commonly occurs in young women
   D requires no surgical treatment

221   Biliary colic typically
   A occurs 3 to 4 hours after meals
   B lasts 5 to 20 minutes
   C radiates from the upper abdomen to the right subscapular region
   D is made worse by deep inspiration

56% on 24/3

218 A **False**   rupture usually occurs between the sixth and twelfth
                   weeks of pregnancy. There is often a history of a
                   missed or scanty menstrual period.
   B **True**   this is associated with vomiting and a desire to
                   defaecate.
   C **True**   a large proportion of patients with this life-threatening
                   condition suffer a rapid and severe blood loss.
   D **True**   a tender cervix and a boggy mass in the vaginal
                   fornices are usually palpable.

219 A **False**   the majority of cases are post-abortal or puerperal.
   B **True**   but other gastrointestinal disturbances are unusual.
   C **False**   this is not a marked feature except in those rare cases
                   which have followed uterine infections.
   D **True**   vaginal examination will reveal this, together with a
                   tender cervix and tenderness in one or other vaginal
                   fornices.

220 A **False**   follicular cyst rupture is the commonest and occurs
                   mid-menstrally. More rarely a luteal cyst may
                   rupture and this will occur premenstrually.
   B **True**   bleeding from the cyst frequently occurs. This causes
                   haemoperitoneum and local peritonitis.
   C **True**
   D **False**   very frequently laparotomy is required to exclude
                   appendicitis. Surgical treatment of the cyst and
                   haemostasis is necessary in a proportion of patients.

221 A **False**   the patient usually gives a past history of dyspepsia,
   B **False**   viz. postprandial flatulence, nausea and epigastric
   C **True**   pain. Biliary colic usually occurs soon after a meal and
   D **True**   lasts at least 3 to 4 hours and often a day or more. The
                   pain is initially felt in the epigastrium or right
                   hypochondrium and later radiates to the back or right
                   subscapular region. It is accentuated by deep
                   breathing.

11 Stomach, duodenum and small intestine

222 **Benign gastric ulcers**
  A occur in the same age group as duodenal ulcers
  B are more common in males than females
  C are more common in the upper social classes
  D produce epigastric pain after eating food

223 **Uncomplicated benign gastric ulcers**
  A occur most commonly on the greater curve of the stomach
  B should initially be treated medically
  C commonly recur after medical treatment
  D should receive surgical treatment if healing has not occured
     after 4 to 6 weeks of medical treatment

224 **Gastric cancer**
  A is more common in males than females
  B is more common in the higher social classes
  C is increasing in frequency in the United Kingdom
  D is more common in rural areas

222 A **False**   they are commoner in older people. The peak
                    incidence for duodenal ulcers is around 30 years
                    whereas gastric ulcers are most common around 50
                    years of age.
     B **True**   the disease is twice as common in men.
     C **False**   there is an increased incidence in the lower social
                    classes.
     D **True**   the pain of gastric ulceration is characteristically felt in
                    the epigastrium and is made worse by eating or
                    drinking strong alcoholic beverages.

223 A **False**   the commonest site is on the lesser curve, particularly
                    around the incisura angularis.
     B **True**   particularly if gastroscopy and endoscopic biopsy
                    indicate that the ulcer is benign.
     C **True**   recurrence rates of as high as 50 per cent have been
                    reported after intensive medical management with
                    antacids, carbenoxolone and bed rest.
     D **True**   if gastroscopic or X-ray evidence of healing has not
                    occurred at the end of this period then surgical
                    treatment (usually a Billroth 1 partial gastrectomy
                    with excision of the ulcer) should be undertaken.
                    These patients are at risk from haemorrhage or
                    perforation. Awareness of the fact that approximately
                    5 per cent of indolent non-healing benign ulcers may
                    be ulcerating cancers masquerading in a benign guise
                    gives further justification to this 'aggressive' approach
                    to treatment.

224 A **True**   throughout the world the incidence in males is
                    approximately twice that of females.
     B **False**   studies from Scandinavia, Japan, USA and the UK all
                    indicate an increased incidence in the lower social
                    classes.
     C **False**   the incidence is decreasing slightly in the UK as in
                    most western countries. This is most striking in the
                    USA where incidence rates in the 1960s were one-
                    third those in the 1930s.
     D **False**   most epidemiological work has shown an increased
                    incidence in urban areas.

225   There is an association of gastric cancer with
   A   achlorhydria of the stomach
   B   atrophic gastritis
   C   adenomatous gastric polyps
   D   duodenal ulceration

226   Surgical treatment of gastric cancer
   A   should preferably be by a total gastrectomy
   B   gives overall 5-year survival figures of 5 to 10 per cent
   C   includes excision of the tumour as a palliative measure
   D   should be advised for all diagnosed cases

227   The signs and symptoms of potentially curable gastric cancer
   A   may simulate those of a benign gastric ulcer
   B   include a hard palpable left supraclavicular node
   C   require investigation by a barium meal examination
   D   require investigation by a gastroscopic examination even
       when the barium meal is normal

225 A **True**   a three- to four-fold increase in incidence has
                      frequently been observed in achlorhydric patients
                      with pernicious anaemia. The majority of patients
                      with gastric cancer have achlorhydria or
                      hypochlorhydria.

   B **True**   long term follow-up of patients with atrophic gastritis
                      has revealed that a higher than expected incidence of
                      gastric cancer is present.

   C **True**   gastric polyps are rare but approximately 20 per cent
                      of them are malignant, especially those which are
                      greater than 2 cm in diameter.

   D **False**   there is no association. Indeed gastric cancer is
                      extremely uncommon in patients with active
                      duodenal ulceration.

226 A **False**   the development of more radical surgical methods to
                      treat stomach cancer has not improved the survival
                      figures except in the case of carcinomas of the cardia.

   B **True**   surgical series do report higher 5-year survival in
                      those patients having gastrectomies but the
                      resectability rate is rarely higher than 70 per cent. The
                      5-year survival rate for patients who had no lymph
                      node metastases at the time of operation is over 40
                      per cent.

? risk of recurrence + malig chance following stomach op

   C **True**   excision is usually more effective palliation than
                      bypass procedures though the mortality is slightly
                      higher.

   D **False**   At least 20 per cent of the patients will present with
                      signs of incurable disease such as a malignant liver
                      enlargement, malignant ascites or a palpable left
                      supraclavicular node. Only necessary palliation
                      should be attempted in these cases.

227 A **True**   pain is the commonest first symptom and may mimic
                      that of gastric or duodenal ulceration. It thus demands
                      a full investigation when appearing in any patient over
                      the age of 50.

   B **False**   neoplastic involvement of Virchow's node is a sign of
                      widespread incurable malignancy originating in the
                      upper gastrointestinal tract.

   C **True**   the diagnostic accuracy of a barium meal for stomach
   D **True**   cancer is approximately 80 per cent. For this reason a
                      negative barium meal in a patient suspected of
                      stomach cancer should be followed by a gastroscopic
                      examination.

228 Gastric cancer
A is most common in the fundus of the stomach
B is most commonly a squamous cell carcinoma
C frequently metastasises via the blood stream
D is most frequently an ulcerating lesion

229 Duodenal diverticulae
A most commonly arise from the concavity of the second part
B are frequently the site of infection, haemorrhage or ulceration
C may be associated with obstructive jaundice
D may follow a severe case of pancreatitis

230 Treatment of symptomatic duodenal ulcers in young patients
A should include twice daily antacids
B should include a strict dietary regime of bland foodstuffs
C should include anti-cholinergic drugs
D should be by early surgery

231 Duodenal ulcers
A have an equal incidence in both sexes
B have a clinical course characterised by long periods of remission
C are characterised by postprandial pain
D occur most commonly in the duodenal cap

228 A **False**   most cancers are situated around the prepyloric and antral regions, especially along the lesser curve.
     B **False**   almost all the carcinomas are adenocarcinomas.
     C **True**   it spreads via the portal blood to produce liver metastases. Systemic blood spread is less common. In addition it may spread by lymphatic permeation, direct extension to neighbouring structures and transcoelomically to produce peritoneal and ovarian metastases.
     D **False**   ulcerating cancers form the minority. The majority have a polypoid form or are diffusely infiltrating (linitis plastica).

229 A **True**   a few may also arise from the third part.
     B **False**   they are only very rarely associated with any
     C **False**   pathology. Though narrow necked diverticulitis is
     D **False**   uncommon and no cases of associated obstructive jaundice have been reported, there are only about 30 cases of rupture of these diverticulae reported therefore elective surgical excision is not advised.

230 A **False**   antacids achieve symptomatic relief by increasing the intragastric pH. However, as this effect does not last longer than 1 hour frequent administration is necessary.
     B **False**   some patients recognise foods that cause exacerbations of pain and avoid those foods. However, in general, dietary control has no part to play in the management of these ulcers.
     C **False**   to be effective in reducing acid output these drugs must be given in doses large enough to be associated with a high incidence of unpleasant side effects. For this reason they are not generally recommended.
     D **False**   duodenal ulcers are extremely common but of very varying severity. Many symptoms are short lived and of minor consequence. The usual indications for surgery are severe and protracted discomfort or complications.

231 A **False**   they are 4 to 5 times more common in males.
     B **True**   this 'periodicity' of the symptoms, wherein remissions alternate with exacerbations lasting from one week to many months, is characteristic.
     C **False**   the epigastric pain generally appears several hours after eating, and thus quite commonly awakes the patient from sleep. It is frequently relieved by food.
     D **True**   95 per cent of ulcers are in the first 1.5 cm of the duodenum (the duodenal cap).

232 Chronic duodenal-ulcers may be treated by
    A histamine H_2-receptor antagonists
    B sub-total gastrectomy
    C vagotomy and gastric drainage
    D highly selective vagotomy (HSV)

233 Acute haemorrhage from a duodenal ulcer
    A requires an urgent barium meal examination
    B requires an urgent gastroscopy
    C should be treated surgically as soon as the diagnosis is made
    D indicates the presence of a chronic duodenal ulcer

234 Post-gastrectomy nutritional disturbances may result in
    A megaloblastic anaemia
    B steatorrhoea
    C iron deficiency anaemia
    D osteoporosis

235 The incidence of Crohn's disease
    A is distributed evenly throughout the world's population
    B is similar in the two sexes
    C is highest amongst young adults
    D is increased in the close relatives of patients of with the
       disease

232 A **True**   a patient with a chronic history, i.e. two or more
                attacks, will always have the tendency to ulceration.
   B **True**   effective long term reduction in acid secretion can be
   C **True**   achieved by an H_2-antagonist or by any of these
   D **True**   operations. Long term medical treatment is often
                indicated in the elderly patient. All the operations
                mentioned will aid ulcer healing. Though subtotal
                gastrectomy has a low recurrent ulcer rate (2–3 per
                cent) its mortality (2 per cent) and high incidence of
                side effects compare unfavourably with vagotomy
                and drainage and HSV. The latter two operations
                account for the majority of operations on duodenal
                ulcer patients at present.

233 A **True**   diagnosis of the source of the haemorrhage should be
   B **True**   sought urgently in order that rational treatment may
                be instituted. These two investigations are
                complementary in achieving this aim.
   C **False** the majority of haemorrhages from duodenal ulcers
                do not require urgent surgery. Surgery is indicated
                when the estimated blood loss is more than 1.5 litres,
                or when there is a second major haemorrhage within
                a few days of the first. Since old poeple stand
                hypovolaemia poorly surgery should be undertaken at
                an earlier stage in this group.
   D **False** acute duodenal ulcers frequently bleed and this is
                particularly common in those associated with major
                burn injury (Curling's ulcer) or multiple injuries.

234 A **True**   megaloblastic anaemia results either from the loss of
                intrinsic factor following excision of the parietal cells
                or vitamin B_{12} deficiency caused by bacterial growth
                in the blind duodenal loop.
   B **True**   this probably results from rapid gastric emptying or
                the food bypassing the duodenum and failing to mix
                with the bile salts in those patients with a
                gastrojejunal anastomosis.
   C **True**   iron deficiency is mainly the result of hypochlorhydria
                and diminshed iron absorption.
   D **True**   this occurs in about 5 per cent of patients, 10 years
                after partial gastrectomy. The reasons are obscure.

235 A **False** it is almost unknown in the tropics. Its incidence is
                highest in the Northern latitudes.
   B **True**   this is apparent at all ages.
   C **True**   the mean age of onset is 25 years, but no age is
                exempt.
   D **True**   between 2 and 6 per cent of cases have been found in
                the family of patients with the disease.

236 Crohn's disease
    A has an infective aetiology
    B is limited to the bowel mucosa
    C does not produce mucosal ulceration
    D is characterised by the absence of fibrous tissue in the
    affected inflamed bowel

237 Patients with Crohn's disease characteristically present with
    A colicky abdominal pain
    B constipation
    C nutritional deficiencies
    D rectal bleeding

238 Systemic manifestations of Crohn's disease include
    A arthralgia
    B finger clubbing
    C growth retardation
    D alopecia

236 A **False**   repeated attempts to identify any infective agent have failed.
     B **False**   lymphoedema is almost always present in the
     C **False**   affected bowel and mesentery — this is associated
     D **False**   with a granulomatous inflammatory process spreading through the whole thickness of the bowel wall. The mucosal surface becomes oedematous and interrupted by longitudinal ulcers producing the typical 'cobblestone' appearance. There is always extensive fibrosis associated with the inflammatory process. This results in the frequent development of stenotic bowel lesions.

237 A **True**   this is the commonest symptom and is related to the increased motility proximal to a partially obstructed bowel.
     B **False**   diarrhoea is almost always present, being the result of partial obstruction, impaired absorption of fluid and bile salts by the diseased bowel, bacterial proliferation in a stagnant loop or any combination of these factors.
     C **True**   bacterial proliferation in stagnant loops of small bowel impairs food absorption, leads to multiple vitamin deficiencies, macrocytic anaemia and steatorrhoea. Loss of weight also results from the anorexia which marks the acute disease.
     D **True**   occult blood loss is almost always present: patients with colonic or rectal Crohn's may well present with rectal bleeding.

238 A **True**   arthralgia and arthritis are commonly associated, particularly in the young patient with Crohn's.
     B **True**   finger clubbing will be found in up to 40 per cent of adults with the disease. It regresses when the disease becomes quiescent.
     C **True**   growth retardation is frequently associated with childhood Crohn's and is associated too with delayed sexual maturation in the presence of normal endrocrimological parameters. It is due to malnutrition resulting from reduced food intake, intestinal blood and protein loss and malabsorption.
     D **False**   there is no recognised association.

239   In the treatment of patients with Crohn's disease
   A   medical methods have no part to play
   B   surgery should be the primary method of treatment
   C   steroids may provide a remission in the progress of the disease
   D   a high bulk diet should be considered

240   Tumours of the small bowel
   A   are rare
   B   may be an inherited disorder
   C   most commonly present with overt or occult rectal bleeding
   D   most commonly present in childhood

239 A **False**   though no drug at present is known to permanently alter the course of the disease, a great improvement can be achieved by supportive measures, e.g. codeine and diphenoxylate will improve the diarrhoea and abdominal cramps; cholestyramine may reduce the faecal water loss by binding bile salts; steatorrhoea may be improved by a low fat diet and antibiotics which deal with the bacteria of a stagnant loop; iron, vitamin B_{12} and folate may be required to deal with anaemia and the use of an elemental diet' or parenteral hyperalimentation may improve the patient's nutrition. Salazopyrine is widely used for long term prophylaxis.

B **False**   though surgery has a large part to play, it is only indicated to deal with the complications such as intestinal obstruction, inflammatory masses or abscesses in the abdomen, internal or external bowel fistulae and indolent anal lesions. Surgery should not be undertaken in the absence of these complications.

C **True**   steroids will induce a remission in the majority of patients and thus have a role in management of the acute case. Prolonged use, however, does not confer further benefit to the patient.

D **False**   this is likely to accentuate those symptoms produced by stenotic bowel lesions.

240 A **True**   they only account for 1 to 2 per cent of all gastrointestinal tumours.

B **True**   intestinal polyposis with melanin pigmentation of the lips, oral mucosa, and palmar and plantar skin is inherited as a Mendelian dominant (Peutz-Jeghers syndrome).

C **False**   intestinal obstruction is more common. This is caused by an intussusception or by the annular intramural spread of a malignant tumour.

D **False**   the majority of patients present after the age of 45 years.

241   Carcinoid tumours of the gastrointestinal tract
   A   are most commonly located in the appendix
   B   are usually malignant
   C   arise in the submucosa
   D   are frequently the cause of gastrointestinal haemorrhage

242   The carcinoid syndrome
   A   characteristically includes abdominal cramps
   B   is produced by the release of vasoconstricting substances
        from the tumour
   C   occurs most commonly with metastatic carcinoid tumours
   D   is usually cured by excision of the primary tumour

243   Chronic radiation injury to the intestinal tract
   A   typically presents with mucosal atrophy
   B   often presents with perforation of the bowel
   C   frequently presents with intestinal obstruction
   D   may present with malabsorption

241 A **True**   whilst they have been found throughout the gastrointestinal tract, the appendix is the commonest site, followed by the small intestine. Bronchial, ovarian and bladder carcinoids also occur.

    B **False**   the majority are benign, particularly those of the appendix. About 30 per cent of small bowel carcinoids do metastasise.

    C **True**   they arise from granular cells in the crypts of Lieberkühn and usually grow submucosally.

    D **False**   mucosal ulceration is uncommon, thus bleeding is rare. A more common complication is intestinal obstruction. Appendiceal carcinoids may initiate luminal obstruction and cause appendicitis.

242 A **True**   these occur together with flushing over the upper half of the body, diarrhoea, wheezing and dyspnoea. The symptoms are often precipitated by food.

    B **False**   vasodilator substances, serotonin, β-hydroxyindoleacetic acid, kallikrein and histamine are released by the tumour.

    C **True**   the appearance of the syndrome nearlly always

    D **False**   indicates hepatic metastases. Although primary carcinoids produce the vasodilator substances, systemic effects are uncommon for they are inactivated on their passage through the liver. Reduction of the tumour burden may improve but not cure the syndrome.

243 A **False**   the injury produces a progressive vasculitis and an associated fibrosis. Epithelial damage, if it occurs, is porbably due to the resultant tissue hypoxia.

    B **True**   the impaired blood supply and progressive fibrosis

    C **True**   result in the intestine becoming thick walled and

    D **True**   stenotic with loops bound to each other by fibrous adhesions. Ulceration and perforation of the bowel may occur. Partial or complete obstruction is common and malabsorption may result from the stagnation of the bowel contents. Surgical excision has a high morbidity and mortality; bypass has rather less. In the absence of severe symptoms supportive medical care is advised.

244   **Acute radiation injury to the intestinal tract**
    A commonly presents with intestinal perforation
    B characteristically produces sloughing of the intestinal mucosa
    C is rarely seen when therapeutic doses of radiation are given to
        the abdomen and pelvis
    D is not seen when the patient is exposed to less than 400 rads

245   **The 'blind-loop' syndrome often**
    A presents with signs of malnutrition
    B presents as a complication of Crohn's disease
    C responds to treatment with oral penicillin
    D shows a reduced excretion of vitamin B_{12} after an
        intramuscular injection of the vitamin

246   **A Meckel's diverticulum of the small intestine**
    A is situated at the jejuno-ileal junction
    B contains all coats of intestinal wall
    C may be associated with a fibrous band connecting it to the
        umbilicus
    D most commonly presents as diverticulitis

66% on 23/B

244 A **False** the most vulnerable cells are those of the mucous
    B **True**   membranes and high doses will result in sloughing of
              the mucosa, haemorrhage and diarrhoea. Perforation
              does not occur in the acute stage but may occur later.
    C **False** nausea, vomiting, intestinal cramps and diarrhoea are
              common when the pelvis is irradiated for carcinoma
              of the cervix or when the abdomen is irradiated in the
              treatment of testicular tumours. These effects subside
              after cessation of therapy and generally require only
              symptomatic relief.
    D **False** the effects of irradiation are related to the size of the
              field to which the body is exposed. 400 rads is the
              LD_{50} for whole body radiation injury. Whole body
              exposure to this and smaller doses may result in
              intestinal injury amongst other effects.

245 A **True**   anaemia, vitamin deficiencies, diarrhoea,
              steatorrhoea and weight loss may result from
              intestinal malabsorption.
    B **True**   any disorder which produces stagnation of bowel
              contents with bacterial overgrowth, such as multiple
              diverticula, strictures or a surgical intestinal bypass
              may produce the 'blind-loop' syndrome.
    C **False** broad spectrum antibiotics which control the
              overgrowth of gram negative organisms are more
              appropriate as a short term form of treatment.
    D **True**   the Schilling test reveals a lower than normal
              excretion of vitamin B_{12} which does not improve with
              the addition of intrinsic factor.

246 A **False** it occurs in the terminal ileum between 50 and 100 cm
              from the ileocaecal valve in 0.5 to 4 per cent of people.
    B **True**   this is a developmental anomaly in which the vitello-
    C **True**   intestinal duct fails to close at its intestinal end. All
              coats of intestinal wall are present and there may also
              be a fibrous cord or, rarely, a fistulous tract between
              the umbilicus and the diverticulum.
    D **False** bleeding due to peptic ulceration arising from
              heterotopic gastric tissue is the commonest
              complication. The next commonest is intestinal
              obstruction usually caused by volvulus of the gut
              around the fibrous band attached to the umbilicus.
              Diverticulitis occurs in less than 25 per cent of
              symptomatic cases. Excision of the diverticulum is
              only recommended in symptomatic cases.

12 Colon, rectum and anus

247 Diverticular disease of the colon
   A   is most common in the tropics
   B   increases in incidence with advancing age
   C   is associated with hypertrophied muscle in the sigmoid colon
   D   is precancerous

248 Diverticular disease of the colon
   A   is usually asymptomatic
   B   often presents with lower abdominal pain
   C   'may present with severe rectal haemorrhage
   D   may present with peritonitis

249 Uncomplicated diverticular disease of the colon
   A   can be most effectively treated with antispasmodics
   B   can be most effectively treated with a high residue diet
   C   frequently requires surgical resection of the sigmoid colon
   D   may require long term antibiotic therapy

247 A **False**   there is a very low incidence in tropical countries.
     B **True**   it is rare below 35 years and the majority of Western people have colonic diverticula by the age of 65.
     C **True**   in diverticular disease higher pressures than usual are developed in the sigmoid colon and this is associated with hypertrophy of the circular muscle coat. Diverticula of mucous membrane develop at sites where blood vessels pierce the muscle wall.
     D **False**   both colonic cancer and diverticular disease are common in Western countries, they therefore frequently coexist. However, no causative relationship has been shown to exist between them.

248 A **True**   uncomplicated and asymptomatic diverticular disease is present in more than half of the population over 50 years of age. Less than 10 per cent of cases are symptomatic.
     B **True**   occlusion of the neck of a diverticulum leads to
     C **True**   inflammation and oedema in the wall of the bowel
     D **True**   which then occludes neighbouring diverticula. The sigmoid colon becomes tender and pericolic inflammation may occur with the formation of abscesses. These may resolve but perforation into the peritoneal cavity, or an adjacent viscus, producing peritonitis or an internal fistula may occur. Occult rectal bleeding is frequently present during these attacks of inflammation and occasionally severe haemorrhage from a vessel in the base of a diverticulum produces massive rectal bleeding.

249 A **False**   there is no antispasmodic agent producing proven
     B **True**   benefit in this disease. Recent evidence suggests that a high bulk diet, containing large amounts of unabsorbed fibre, will increase the faecal bulk, reduce the colonic pressures and halt the progression of the pathological process.
     C **False**   surgery should be reserved for the complications of diverticular disease and those cases in which the diagnosis of colonic cancer cannot be excluded.
     D **False**   there is no evidence that prophylactic antibiotics will reduce the attacks of inflammation.

250   In ulcerative colitis
  A the colonic mucosa demonstrates multiple wide ulcers and inflammatory changes
  B there is extensive fibrosis of the colonic wall
  C colonic pseudopolyps are a feature of the early stages of the disease
  D extensive inflammatory changes also occur in the ileum

251   In patients with ulcerative colitis a barium enema examination
  A should not be performed unless the disease is quiescent
  B often demonstrates a smooth and thinned colon
  C is of value in confirming the presence of proctitis
  D is necessary for the patients' future medical or surgical management

252.   Surgical treatment of ulcerative colitis
  A is usually by subtotal colectomy
  B is usually undertaken as an urgent measure
  C may reduce the risk of colonic cancer
  D is often indicated for colitis confined to the rectosigmoid region

250 A **True**   this is the fundamental pathological change, the
                   aetiology of which is unknown.

   B **False**   repeated attacks of inflammation thin the mucosal
                  surface and extend the inflammatory process into the
                  muscularis mucosae and eventually the muscular
                  layers of the colonic walls. Fibrosis, resulting in
                  shortening and stricture formation, may then occur.

   C **False**   pseudopolyps are the result of repeated attacks of
                  inflammation and ulceration and may be regarded as
                  abnormal regeneration of colonic mucosa.

   D **False**   much attention was given to an associated mild ileitis
                  and it was thought that this represented an extension
                  of the colonic disease to the small bowel. It is now
                  thought more likely that it results from backwash of
                  abnormal colonic contents through an incompetent
                  ileocaecal valve.

251 A **False**   though it is dangerous to perform this examination in
                   patients suffering from acute and severe forms of the
                   disease it can be performed safely at other times.

   B **True**   lack of haustration and a decreased colonic calibre
   C **False**   indicate chronic colitis. It is usually difficult to
   D **True**   estimate the extent of mucosal ulceration and
                  inflammation particularly of the rectum. The
                  demonstration of chronic colitis with stenotic areas or
                  suspected carcinoma is helpful when considering
                  future management.

252 A **False**   total proctocolectomy and permanent ileostomy is the
                   most usual choice of operation, though a case can be
                   made out for rectal preservation if it is not severely
                   affected. In such cases careful observation of the
                   rectal stump is obligatory to avoid the risk of cancer
                   becoming established.

   B **False**   elective surgery is the general rule. Toxic dilatation of
                  the colon, acute perforation and severe haemorrhage
                  necessitate emergency surgery but fortunately these
                  complications are rare.

   C **True**   in total colitis there is a cumulative risk of colonic
                  cancer developing—initially the risk is low but after 20
                  years of the disease it rises at 5 per cent per annum.
                  After 25 years there is a 40 per cent risk of developing
                  cancer, thus prophylactic colectomy is being more
                  frequently under taken in long-standing cases.

   D **False**   less than 5 per cent of these cases require colonic
                  operations. There is no increased risk of malignant
                  change developing in this form of the disease.

253   Long term medical management of ulcerative colitis
    A   is usually indicated in patients with total colonic involvement
    B   is usually indicated in children
    C   is effective in the majority of patients
    D   includes intravenous pitressin in acute exacerbations

254   Ulcerative colitis
    A   is more common in males than females
    B   appears most commonly between the ages of 20 and 30
    C   usually presents with abdominal discomfort and diarrhoea
    D   can usually be diagnosed on sigmoidoscopic examination

255   Crohn's disease of the rectum
    A   is associated with an anal fissure or fistula in the majority of cases
    B   may produce a diffuse granular proctitis
    C   is usually associated with ileal or colonic Crohn's disease
    D   is characterised by long periods of remission

256   Ischaemic colitis
    A   often presents with diarrhoea
    B   often presents with rectal bleeding
    C   is commonly situated around the splenic flexure
    D   is often effectively managed by non-surgical means

253 A **False**   children, the aged, patients with total colonic
     B **False**   involvement and those patients with severe attacks
     C **True**   are all in a 'high risk' category wherein relapses are
     D **False**   frequent. Medical management is generally
                     unsatisfactory in these groups of patients. The
                     remainder can be managed medically with
                     symptomatic measures such as sedatives,
                     anti-diarrhoeal drugs, vitamins and iron.
                     Sulphasalazine should be used as maintenance
                     therapy. It has been shown to reduce the incidence of
                     relapse. Steroid enemata are of use in the acute attack
                     and these may be supplemented by systemic steroids
                     or ACTH for a short time.

254 A **False**   there is an increased incidence in females (1.5 : 1).
     B **True**   though the majority of patients present in early adult
                     life, increasing numbers of patients are now
                     presenting in old age.
     C **True**   these two symptoms together with rectal bleeding are
                     by far the most common. Fever, joint effusions and
                     pain, uveitis and erythema nodosum are associated
                     symptoms in a minority of cases.
     D **True**   almost all cases of ulcerative colitis have an
                     associated proctitis, and sigmoidoscopy shows a
                     granular oedematous mucosa which is friable and
                     bleeds easily. Rectal biopsies will confirm the
                     diagnosis.

255 A **True**   three-quarters of these patients have one of these
                     lesions.
     B **True**   but the granulomatous infiltration of the submucosa
                     more frequently causes patchy mucosal nodularity
                     and ulceration.
     C **True**   isolated rectal involvement is rarely encountered.
     D **False**   the disease is progressive, in contrast to nonspecific
                     proctitis.

256 A **False**   diarrhoea is not an early feature. The ischaemic
     B **True**   mucosa becomes oedematous and ulcerates. This
                     produces significant blood loss into the bowel lumen
                     and lower abdominal pain. The pathogenesis is
                     frequently obscure for often no occlusion can be
                     found in the appropriate colonic vessels.
     C **True**   though all parts of the colon may be affected the
                     splenic flexure is the area most commonly involved.
     D **True**   many patients may be managed by close observation,
                     blood and fluid replacement and antibiotic therapy. A
                     barium enema will demonstrate localised oedema of
                     the bowel wall in the early stages. Late ischaemic
                     strictures may develop and require surgical relief.

257   Acute volvulus of the sigmoid colon
    A most frequently occurs in Eastern Europe and Africa
    B is relatively common amongst athletes
    C usually produces abdominal distension which is most marked
       on the left side
    D may be effectively treated without resorting to laparotomy

258   Hirschsprung's disease
    A is the result of acquired aganglionosis of the large bowel
    B usually becomes evident in early adult life
    C can usually be diagnosed on a barium enema
    D can usually be managed by dietary means

257 A **True**   there is a high incidence in the Western World
amongst institutionalised patients, but the highest
rates are reported from Eastern Europe and Africa
where high bulk diets have been blamed for
producing colonic distension. Only 15 per cent of
cases involve the caecum. Most of the remainder
occur in the sigmoid colon where a redundant loop
usually rotates on the sigmoid mesocolon.

   B **False**   there is no relation.

   C **True**   the patient presents with colicky lower abdominal
pain, vomiting and gross asymmetrical distension of
the abdomen. In sigmoid volvulus this is maximal on
the left side.

   D **True**   unless these are signs of colonic strangulation the
patient should be placed in the knee–elbow position
(this may itself untwist the loop) and sigmoidoscoped,
after which a flatus tube is gently introduced into the
twisted loop to decompress. Failure to achieve this
satisfying result indicates that surgical reduction or
resection is required.

258 A **False**   this is congenital condition in which aganglionosis of
the rectum and part of the colon results in lack of
peristaltic activity and some degree of large bowel
obstruction.

   B **False**   most patients with this complaint have some degree
of constipation in the neonatal period. Only a few
cases will present in later life.

   C **True**   the barium enema reveals dilatation of the normal
colon proximal to the aganglionic segment which is of
normal diameter. Diagnosis can be confirmed by a
rectal biopsy which reveals the absence of a
myenteric nerve plexus.

   D **False**   resection or bypass of the aganglionic segment must
be performed. This is frequently preceded by a
colostomy.

259   Colonic polpys
   A   are associated with colonic cancer
   B   may be hereditary
   C   should not be removed if they are asymptomatic
   D   are usually hyperplastic

260   Villous papillomata of the large bowel
   A   are usually sessile
   B   are more common on the right side of the colon
   C   may cause renal failure
   D   rarely become malignant

261   A right-sided colonic cancer frequently presents with
   A   anaemia
   B   intestinal obstruction
   C   rectal bleeding
   D   an abdominal mass

259 A **True**   in 10 per cent of resected colonic cancers there are
neighbouring benign polyps. There is good
epidiomological evidence to support the view that
adenomatous polyps are precancerous.

  B **True**   familial polyposis is inherited as a Mendelian
dominant. It is a premalignant condition and
neoplasia can only be avoided by total colectomy
before the age of 20.

  C **False**   polyps occur in 10 to 20 per cent of the adult
population and many are symptomless. However,
neoplasia will arise in a proportion of polyps,
therefore those that are sessile, greater than 2 cm,
bleeding or apparently infiltrating should be removed
as a prophylactic measure.

  D **False**   adenomatous polyps are the commonest tumours but
juvenile polyps and hyperplastic polyps are not
infrequently encountered.

260 A **True**   these are velvety soft polypoid tumours which
  B **False**   frequently spread to surround the bowel lumen. Areas
of malignant change can be recognised by surface
ulceration or areas of induration. 90 per cent of the
tumours occur in the rectum and distal half of the
sigmoid colon.

  C **True**   occasionally the loss of mucus from these tumours is
so excessive (amounting to 3 litres or more per day)
that hypokalaemia, hyponatraemia, dehydration and
renal failure occur.

  D **False**   whilst the majority of these tumours are benign, they
have a very high malignant potential. Invasive
carcinoma has been reported in up to 40 per cent of
these lesions.

261 A **True**   the general pattern of symptomatology of right sided
  B **False**   colonic cancers is determined by (i) their relatively
  C **False**   long distance from the anus, and (ii) the fluid bowel
  D **True**   contents of the right side of the colon. Bleeding does
occur from these cancers but it is well mixed with the
stool, frequently passing unnoticed by the patient
until anaemia is present. Because the bowel contents
of the right colon are fluid, intestinal obstruction is
rare and the tumour frequently enlarges to become
palpable or indeed visible on abdominal examination.

262   A left-sided colonic cancer frequently presents with
    A   anaemia
    B   intestinal obstruction
    C   rectal bleeding
    D   abdominal pain

263   Curative cancer surgery of the colon necessitates
    A   total excision of all neoplastic tissue
    B   excision of all neighbouring related lymph nodes in continuity
    C   early control of the arterial supply to the tumour to prevent
          blood-borne metastases during manipulation
    D   a routine 'second look' laparotomy to detect and treat early
          recurrence

264   Surgical excision of a colonic cancer
    A   is the only mode of cure
    B   may be inferior in terms of cure rate to radiotherapy
    C   should not be attempted in the presence of widespread
          metastases
    D   is complicated by anastomotic recurrences

262 A **False**   the left side of the colon is narrower than the right,
    B **True**   nearer to the anus and its contents are more solid,
    C **True**   thus rectal bleeding is usually overt and noticed by the
    D **True**   patient. The tumour frequently causes a degree of
                   obstruction which produces lower abdominal pain
                   and pencil like stools or frank obstruction. Thus the
                   presentation of patients with left sided cancers is
                   frequently earlier than patients with right sided
                   cancers. Anaemia is a less common presentation in
                   left sided lesions.

263 A **True**   in order to remove the likeliest foci of spread of
    B **True**   malignant cells.
    C **False**   in order to diminish the potential risk of tumour cell
                  embolisation the veins draining the region of the
                  growth are ligated before mobilisation of the
                  malignancy begins. Arterial ligation can have no such
                  benefit.
    D **False**   this procedure, though it possesses theoretical
                  advantages, is not yet widely used. It remains to be
                  demonstrated whether any improvement in survival is
                  sufficient to outweigh the morbidity and mortality of
                  the second procedure.

264 A **True**   it succeeds in curing 70 per cent of cases where the
                  tumour is confined to the bowel wall and 30 per cent
                  of those where lymph node metastases are noted.
    B **False**   radiotherapy is used in some centres as an adjunct to
                  surgery for rectal cancer but the adenocarcinoma is
                  relatively insensitive to radiation. It is not possible to
                  safely give curative doses of radiation to the intestinal
                  tract.
    C **False**   removal of an obstructing, bleeding, painful lesion is
                  in most cases the most effective palliation for
                  incurable cancer of the colon.
    D **True**   intraluminal scatter of neoplastic cells is increased
                  during surgical manipulation of the bowel, which may
                  be the cause of the anastamotic recurrences. It is
                  likely, however, that these are due to residual tumour
                  in the surgical field.

265   The survival of treated patients with large bowel cancer depends on
- A   the absence of lymph node metastasis
- B   the degree of differentiation of the cancer
- C   whether the primary is right or left sided
- D   the involvement of other organs

266   The early diagnosis of rectal cancer may be most reliably achieved by
- A   rectal and sigmoidoscopic examination
- B   barium enema examination
- C   faecal occult blood estimations
- D   detailed investigation of all patients with iron deficiency anaemia

267   Rectal cancer
- A   is usually of squamous cell origin
- B   usually metastasises by lymphatic spread
- C   frequently presents with faecal impaction
- D   frequently requires a barium enema for accurate diagnosis

268   Rectal bleeding
- A   which is bright red and occurring on defaecation is usually arising from the anal canal
- B   which is dark and mixed with the stool is arising from the rectum or above
- C   should be investigated by a sigmoidoscopic examination in all cases
- D   should be investigated by a barium enema examination in all cases

265 A **True**   the status of the lymph nodes is a most important
     B **True**   determinant of survival, for when cancer is present in
     C **True**   the nodes, the survival rate drops to half that of a
     D **True**   comparable tumour whithout nodes. Anaplastic
                      tumours have the worst prognosis and the prognosis
                      worsens if the tumour has spread through the bowel
                      wall, particularly if it spreads extraserosally to involve
                      other organs. There appears to be an improved
                      survival in comparable right-sided tumours—
                      possibly due to the relative ease with which radical
                      resection can be performed.

266 A **True**   50 per cent of all large bowel tumours lie within reach
                      of the sigmoidoscope and half of these are palpable
                      by the examining finger.
     B **False**   the capacious rectum does not readily yield its secrets
                      to the radiogist—a sigmoidoscopy is essential before
                      this investigation.
     C **False**   benign causes of faecal blood loss are very common.
     D **True**   this will include full investigation of the
                      gastrointestinal tract including sigmoidoscopy and
                      possibly a barium enema examination.

267 A **False**   the vast majority are adenocarcinomata.
     B **True**   lymphatic spread to pararectal and inferior mesenteric
                      nodes is common. Venous spread also occurs and
                      results in liver metastases.
     C **False**   obstruction is a very rare symptom in this condition. It
                      usually presents with rectal bleeding, the passage of
                      slime rectally or a sensation of constant rectal
                      fullness.
     D **False**   many of the neoplasms can be palpated by digital
                      examination. Barium enema examinations will
                      demonstrate associated colonic pathology but are
                      imprecise in the examination of the rectum.

268 A **True**   in these cases the blood is not mixed with the stool.
     B **True**   decomposition of the blood and some mixing with the
                      stool occurs when bleeding is from the rectum or
                      above.
     C **True**   if the history suggests anal canal bleeding and
     D **False**   proctosigmoidoscopy confirms this and verifies that
                      there is no other cause in the lowest 25 cm of the
                      gastrointestinal tract then barium enema need not be
                      undertaken. However, a barium enema is necessary if
                      the sigmoidoscopy is normal.

269 Internal haemorrhoids
   A usually cause pruritis
   B Are often associated with intense pain
   C often become infected
   D will often resolve after conservative treatment

270 An anal fistula
   A is usually a congenital condition
   B often presents with pruritis
   C may be associated with chronic colonic inflammation
   D can be successfully treated with a low residue diet

271 An anal fissure
   A is an ulcer of the anal mucosa
   B usually lies anteriorly
   C is more common in men
   D can usually, in acute cases be treated conservatively

272 Perianal abscesses
   A commence in the anal wall
   B have the same aetiology as ischiorectal abscesses
   C are effectively treated by antibiotics
   D may result in a fistula-in-ano

269 A **True**   they cause prolapse and thus produce irritation of the anal skin. Some mucous discharge follows and the perianal skin becomes excoriated and pruritic.

B **False**   uncomplicated internal haemorrhoids are usually painless. Internal haemorrhoidal thrombosis produces severe anal pain which may not be relieved until haemorrhoidectomy is performed. External haemorrhoidal thrombosis is common and very painful for 3 to 5 days.

C **False**   this is an unusual complication.

D **True**   attention to bowel habit by the prescription of a high bulk diet will help minor haemorrhoids to regress.

270 A **False**   this is an acquired condition usually arising from infected anal glands.

B **True**   the discharging sinus results in maceration of the perianal skin and pruritis.

C **True**   30 per cent of patients with colonic Crohn's disease also possess anal fissures of fistulae. There is a high incidence also in chronic ulcerative colitis.

D **False**   only surgical excision of all the sinus tract will result in cure.

271 A **True**   it is a linear ulcer of the anal canal usually lying
B **False**   posteriorly. Constipation is a common cause, it causes
C **False**   intense pain during defaecation and is more common in women.

D **True**   the majority of acute fissures will heal with a laxative and local anaesthetic cream but if this fails a firm digital stretch under anaesthesia is usually curative. It is important to remember that the condition is common in Crohn's disease and that it may be confused with a squamous cell cancer of the anal canal.

272 A **True**   both ischiorectal and perianal abscesses usually arise
B **True**   from intersphincteric abscesses arising from infected anal glands.

C**False**   antibiotics will not resolve established abscesses; early incision and drainage is required.

D **True**   if the infection does not completely resolve, it is likely that a fistula-in-ano will result.

273   Rectal prolapse
  A is commonly seen in infants
  B is commonly seen in the elderly
  C is often associated with poor anal tone
  D may in some cases be successfully treated by
     haemorrhoidectomy

274   Carcinoma of the anus
  A is generally an adenocarcinoma
  B readily spreads to the inguinal lymph nodes
  C has a similar prognosis to rectal carcinoma
  D should usually be treated by an abdominoperineal resection
     of rectum

273 A **True**   the disease commonly occurs in both age groups. It is
     B **True**   particularly common amongst elderly childless
                    women. In infants it is fortunately not a chronic
                    condition.
     C **True**   this is most usual in the elderly and is associated with
                    faecal incontinence.
     D **True**   for mild degrees of prolapse in the elderly a mucosal
                    resection is sufficient treatment; other patients may
                    need the insertion of a Thiersch wire around the anus;
                    occasionally some form of rectal fixation is required.

274 A **False**   squamous cell carcinoma is far more common.
     B **True**   it reaches these nodes via the lymphatics of the
                    perianal skin.
     C **True**   there is an overall 5-years survival rate of 40 per cent
                    in both neoplasms.
     D **True**   this allows wide excision of the perianal lymphatics.
                    The inguinal nodes should be carefully observed and
                    excised if metastases are suspected.

13 The liver

275 **Bile**
- A is secreted by the liver only after the ingestion of food
- B is secreted at the rate of 200 to 400 ml per day
- C secretion is reduced after cholecystectomy
- D contains cholecystokinin

276 **Bilirubin**
- A is synthesised from cholesterol
- B is conjugated in the liver
- C is excreted into the bowel where it forms urobilinogen
- D may be formed from reabsorbed urobilinogen

277 **A patient with chronic liver failure characteristically presents with**
- A tremors
- B disorders of consciousness
- C palmar erythema
- D a cold collapsed peripheral circulation

278 **The diagnosis of chronic liver disease may be helped by serum estimations of**
- A alkaline phosphatase
- B creatine phosphokinase
- C glutamic pyruvic transaminase (SGPT)
- D glutamic oxaloacetic transaminase (SGOT)

275 A **False** the liver continually secretes bile at the rate of 600 to
    B **False** 800ml/day. Food intake has very little effect on biliary
      secretion.
    C **False** the gallbladder performs a storage function and is
      non-secretory. Its removal does not affect the biliary
      secretion of the liver.
    D **False** this intestinal hormone is released by the duodenal
      mucosa after the entry of food into the duodenum. It
      causes the gallbladder to contract and the sphincter of
      Oddi to relax.

276 A **False** it is formed from the breakdown of haemoglobin by
      cells of the reticulo-endothelial system.
    B **True** it is transported, bound to albumin, to the liver and
      there combined with glucuronic acid to form
      conjugated bilirubin.
    C **True** conjugated bilirubin is broken down by intestinal
      bacteria to form urobilinogen.
    D **True** half of the urobilinogen is reabsorbed from the
      intestinal tract and reconverted to bilirubin in the liver.

277 A **True** there is a coarse tremor of voluntary muscle, in
      advanced liver failure.
    B **True** this ranges from confusion to coma. It is exacerbated
      by a high protein intake or a gastrointestinal bleed
      because of the rise in the circulating undetoxicated
      protein products.
    C **True** vasomotor tone is decreased, all peripheral pulses are
    D **False** easily felt and the extremities are warmer and more
      erythematous than normal.

278 A **True** this enzyme is produced by bone and excreted in the
      bile. Therefore both bone and hepatobiliary diseases
      may produce a rise in its normal value.
    B **False** this enzyme is increased in the serum after muscle
      damage.
    C **True** both these enzymes are widely distributed but
    D **True** particularly highly concentrated in the liver. Acute
      liver damage thus produces a rise in their serum
      levels.

279   Liver failure
A   is the most common cause of death in patients who present with bleeding oesophageal varices
B   may be precipitated by diuretics in cirrhotic patients
C   may present with personality changes
D   can be effectively treated on a temporary basis by haemodialysis

280   The ascites of chronic liver failure may be due to
A   hypoalbuminaemia
B   increased aldosterone secretion
C   hepatic vein obstruction
D   portal vein occlusion

281   The anaemia associated with chronic liver disease may be due to
A   gastrointestinal bleeding
B   decreased red cell survival
C   hypersplenism
D   deficiency of intrinsic factor

282   Bleeding oesophageal varices
A   can be reliably diagnosed from a barium swallow examination
B   may be treated by an oesophageal transection
C   may be treated by a portocaval shunt
D   are best treated by injection sclerotherapy

279 A **True**   the commonest cause of death is liver failure whether the varices are medically or surgically treated.

B **True**   disorders of fluid and electrolyte balance, particularly the hypokalaemia induced by most diuretics, may precipitate hepatic coma.

C **True**   in the early stages alteration in mood is noted but this progresses to disorientation, stupor and finally coma. Associated with these signs are a coarse tremor, warm extremities and a mousy odour on the breath.

D **False**   all treatment is supportive and aimed at reducing the nitrogenous content of the bowel while maintaining fluid and electrolyte balance. There is no evidence that haemodialysis, exchange transfusion or liver perfusion achieves better results.

280 A **True**   all these factors play a part but the most important is
B **True**   hepatic venous obstruction and the raised
C **True**   intrahepatic pressures that follow. Ascites rarely
D **True**   follows an isolated portal vein occlusion.

281 A **True**   gastrointestinal bleeding from either oesophageal
B **True**   varices or duodenal ulceration is common in
C **True**   cirrhotics. There is also a decreased red cell survival time. Hypersplenism often accompanies the splenic enlargement of portal hypertension and results in a depression of all blood elements.

D **False**   this is not present.

282 A **False**   the history of painless vomiting of large quantities of fresh blood leads to an accurate diagnosis in most cases. Barium swallow and meal should be performed and will reveal positive evidence of varices in over 90 per cent of affected patients. Oesophagogastroscopy is essential to demonstrate whether the varices are the cause of the haemorrhage.

B **True**   transection will stop variceal bleeding for a period of
C **True**   time but bleeding tends to recur earlier than when a portocaval shunt is undertaken. The surgical mortality is similar in both procedures, being about 40 per cent.

D **True**   effective injection of sclerosant is possible via the flexible gastroscope. Bleeding can be controlled with a much lower immediate mortality. Injection may need to be repeated in a few months time.

283   **Portal hypertension**
    A is due to extrahepatic causes in approximately 50 per cent of
       cases
    B most commonly presents in the third decade
    C which is associated with cirrhosis is due to post-sinusoidal
       obstruction
    D does not usually affect life expectancy

284   **Emergency management of bleeding oesophageal varices
      should include**
    A frequent enemas
    B infusions of hypertonic saline
    C large quantities of intravenous potassium
    D intravenous posterior pituitary extract

285   **The Sengstaken triple lumen double balloon tube**
    A should be routinely used in the management of bleeding
       oesophageal varices
    B has significantly reduced the mortality rate of oesophageal
       haemorrhage.
    C has relatively few complications in use
    D is a more effective haemostatic appliance when the balloons
       are inflated with very cold liquids

286   **Splenoportography**
    A should be performed under a general anaesthetic
    B allows portal pressure to be estimated
    C may demonstrate the site of portal vein obstruction
    D is helpful in the diagnosis of hepatic tumours

283 A **False**   intrahepatic causes due to cirrhosis account for 90 per cent of cases. The major extrahepatic cause is portal vein thrombosis.

   B **False**   cirrhosis takes many years to develop and thus the majority of patients are in late middle life.

   C **True**   the cirrhotic process particularly constricts the smallest tributaries of the hepatic veins.

   D **False**   the 5-year survival is very poor; only 5 to 10 per cent of patients with cirrhosis and portal hypertension survive this period.

284 A **True**   together with oral neomycin and nasogastric aspiration these will reduce the risk of hepatic coma arising from bacterial action on the nitrogenous bowel contents.

   B **False**   fresh blood will almost certainly be required. Cirrhotic patients have a marked increase in total body sodium and thus saline infusions should only be given after exceptional losses.

   C **True**   hypokalaemic alkalosis frequently accompanies bleeding oesophageal varices.

   D **True**   this produces a temporary drop in portal pressure, sufficient in some cases to stop the bleeding.

285 A **True**   this tube has a limited role in providing a very
   B **False**   temporary means of stopping massive haemorrhage
   C **False**   prior to surgery. Rebleeding frequently follows withdrawal of the balloon. Oesophageal perforation, aspiration pneumonia and asphyxia have been reported after its use.

   D **False**   it is not possible to circulate fluid through these balloons and it is unlikely that local hypothermia stops gastro-oesophageal bleeding.

286 A **False**   the technique is usually performed under local anaesthesia via a needle introduced percutaneously into the splenic pulp.

   B **True**   there is a close correlation between the splenic pulp pressure and that in the portal vein. In health this varies between 8 and 12 cm of water.

   C **True**   it may differentiate between intra-and extra-hepatic causes of portal hypertension.

   D **True**   Space occupying lesions of the liver are well demonstrated by the abnormal intrahepatic venous pattern but this use of the investigations has been superceded by ultrasound and CAT scans.

287   A portocaval shunt

A   should, where possible, be performed in patients with
oesophageal varices before bleeding occurs
(prophylactically)

B   carries the risk of precipitating liver failure.

C   prevents further haemorrhage from varices in the large
majority of patients

D   is most applicable to cases with extrahepatic portal occlusion

288   A liver abscess

A   is commonly associated with gallstones

B   typically produces a firm enlarged tender liver

C   is usually accompanied by jaundice

D   commonly produces a right sided pleural effusion

289   Hydatid cysts of the liver

A   are frequently asymptomatic

B   are commoner in Australia

C   require surgical removal

D   may produce jaundice and fever

287 A **False**   there is no evidence to suggest that this form of
                     'prophylactic' shunt surgery improves longevity.
                     However, once the varices have bled then successful
                     shunt surgery is followed by a 5-year survival of
                     approximately 50 per cent of patients. 'Medical'
                     management of this group results in almost 100·per
                     cent mortality over the same period.

   B **True**   liver failure is the commonest major complication
   C **True**   after shunt surgery, and may result in death.
                     Rebleeding however does not commonly occur.

   D **False**   this rare cause of portal hypertension can only be
                     treated by a splenorenal or mesocaval portosystemic
                     anastomosis.

288 A **True**   the commonest cause in Britain of a liver abscess is
   B **True**   cholangitis associated with gallstones in the common
   C **True**   bile duct. The patient is pyrexial with pain in the right
   D **True**   upper quadrant due to an enlarged tender liver.
                     Jaundice is almost always present and an ipsilateral
                     pleural effusion is common. X-rays show elevation of
                     the diaphragm, blood cultures are frequently positive
                     and ultrasonography or liver scanning may
                     demonstrate the lesion. Antibiotics and surgical
                     drainage are required.

289 A **True**   in its life cycle, the echinococcus has dog as its
   B **True**   primary host and sheep, cattle or man as its
                     intermediate host. Thus the disease is commoner in
                     rural areas. Infestation occurs by the ingested
                     embryos passing through the portal vein to the liver
                     where they reproduce to form multilocular cysts—
                     many of which are asymptomatic.

   C **True**   once the diagnosis is confirmed (by X-rays, liver
   D **True**   scans, Casoni and other serological tests) the cyst
                     should be removed for rupture of the cyst may occur
                     and cause fever, jaundice and possibly anaphylactic
                     shock due to the dissemination of multiple daughter
                     cysts.

290   **Liver cancer**
    A   is commoner in patients with cirrhosis
    B   often presents with ascites
    C   has an increased incidence in sheep farmers
    D   produces measurable serum levels of a fetal protein

291   **Liver metastases**
    A   commonly arise from gastrointestinal neoplasms
    B   occur only by tumour embolisation of the portal vein
    C   may be palliated by hepatic artery ligation
    D   are usually seminecrotic

290 A **True**   about 5 per cent of all cirrhotics will develop liver
                   cancer, and cirrhotics account for 75 per cent of all
                   liver cancers.

   B **True**   the presentation is sudden, with rapidly progressive
                   ascites, weight loss, jaundice and pain in the right
                   hypochondrium.

   C **False**   hydatid disease, but not liver cancer, is commoner in
                   sheep farmers.

   D **True**   all the liver function tests may be abnormal,
                   particularly the alkaline phosphatase. Alpha
                   fetoprotein is noted in more than 50 per cent of the
                   patients with primary liver cancer.

291 A **True**   but bloodspread from lung, breast and kidney
                   neoplasms are frequently seen.

   B **False**   portal vein emboli are a cause but they commonly
                   result from emboli carried by the hepatic artery.

   C **True**   this appears to be the cause — but whilst relief of
                   symptoms may follow there has been no
                   demonstration of any benefit in long term survival.

   D **False**   though they appear umbilicated with soft centres they
                   frequently have a sufficient blood supply to allow
                   massive growth to occur.

14 Extrahepatic biliary system, spleen and pancreas

292 Acute cholecystitis
A is almost invariably related to the presence of gallstones
B usually presents with biliary colic
C is often associated with jaundice
D is characterised by a pyrexia in the early hours of the disease

293 Chronic cholecystitis
A may cause persistent epigastric discomfort
B can occur in the presence of a normal cholecystogram
C may be premalignant
D may be effectively treated medically

294 Acute cholecystitis should usually be treated by
A nasogastric suction and intravenous fluids
B antibiotic therapy
C urgent cholecystectomy
D cholecystostomy

292 A **True**   more than 95 per cent of the patients with acute
                       cholecystitis have gallstones. Acute cholecystitis
                       usually follows blockage of the cystic duct with a
                       stone.

     B **True**   the pain is felt in the right upper quadrant and often
                       radiates to the back, becoming continuous in 2 or 3
                       hours. Reflex vomiting is usually present.

     C **True**   a slightly raised bilirubin (about 2 to 3 mg/100ml (30 to
                       45 μmol/1)) is frequently found in acute cholecystitis.
                       Bilirubin values above this level usually indicate a
                       stone in the common bile duct.

     D **False**   cystic duct calculus obstruction often relieves itself
                       before the distended gallbladder becomes
                       secondarily infected. Where this does not occur
                       cholecystitis develops and pyrexia develops after 24
                       to 36 hours.

293 A **False**   the pain is intermittent, colicky and often
                       post-prandial.

     B **False**   poor opacification, non-opacification or the presence
                       of gallstones are always noted.

     C **True**   gallbladder cancer though rare always occurs in the
                       chronically inflamed gallbladder. This may be a
                       justification for elective removal of such inflamed
                       bladders in the relatively young and fit patient but is
                       rarely so in the elderly frail patient.

     D **True**   medical dissolution of cholesterol gallstones by bile
                       acids is occasionally possible providing they are small
                       radiolucent and lying in a 'functioning' gallbladder.

294 A **True**   the majority of cases will respond to conservative
     B **True**   treatment. This is followed by an elective
     C **False**   cholecystectomy, 2 or 3 months later. However, an
     D **False**   increasing number of surgeons believe urgent
                       cholecystectomy to be desirable in that it prevents
                       recurrence of infection which is not uncommon in the
                       waiting period. Cholecytostomy is only occasionally
                       indicated when acute cholecystitis does not resolve
                       after conservative management and cholecystectomy
                       is judged too hazardous.

295   Biliary obstruction
   A   may be diagnosed by decreased bromsulphthalein (BSP) clearance
   B   may be diagnosed by decreased biliary excretion of rose bengal dye
   C   may be diagnosed by an oral cholecystogram
   D   may cause a prolonged prothrombin time

296   Gallstones
   A   have an incidence which increases with age
   B   are more frequent in females
   C   usually contain a predominance of calcium carbonate
   D   are formed in bile which is supersaturated with bile acids

297   Cholesterol gallstones
   A   are the commonest type of gallstones in the Western World
   B   usually occur in patients with abnormalities of bile composition
   C   may form in the common bile duct
   D   may undergo dissolution after protracted therapy with bile acids

295 A **False**   BSP is cleared from the blood by the liver and the test is used to appraise hepatocellular function. The presence of biliary obstruction invalidates the investigation.

   B **True**   this synthetic dye is cleared from the blood stream by the liver and excreted in the bile. When labelled with 1^{131} its excretion can be estimated by radiation counters.

   C **False**   the contrast media are not concentrated in the bile when the serum bilirubin is above 3 mg/100 ml (51 μmol/1) and so no radiological diagnosis is possible by this technique.

   D **True**   the lack of bile salts in the intestinal tract interferes with the absorption of vitamin K_1 which is essential for prothrombin synthesis. This defect may be overcome by an intramuscular injection of vitamin K_1.

296 A **True**   15 to 20 per cent of adults over the age of 40 have
   B **True**   gallstones. Females are much more commonly affected than males, particularly in middle life.

   C **False**   the majority of stones have cholesterol as their major component. It is mixed with calcium carbonate and bilirubinate.

   D **False**   gallstones tend to form in abnormal bile which is supersaturated with cholesterol or with calcium bilirubinate.

297 A **True** F   75 per cent of 'Western' gallstones are predominantly cholesterol containing. but not just cholesterol

   B **True**   the bile is saturated or supersaturated with cholesterol.

   C **True**   though 90 per cent of such stones are formed in the gallbladder they can form in the biliary tree.

   D **True**   cholesterol stones which are small radio-opaque and within the gallbladder may be dissolved after 6 to 9 months of such therapy but reform frequently once treatment ceases.

298   The presence of stones in the common bile duct
   A   is commonly associated with a long history of dyspepsia
   B   is invariably associated with jaundice
   C   must be considered during every cholecystectomy
   D   occasionally requires treatment by
          choledochoduodenostomy

299   Stones in the common bile duct
   A   are present in nearly 50 per cent of cases of cholecystitis
   B   often give rise to jaundice, fever and biliary colic
   C   are usually accompanied by progressive jaundice
   D   are not usually associated with a distended gallbladder

300   Oral cholecystography
   A   may not opacify the gallbladder when gallstones are present
   B   is frequently unsatisfactory if intestinal absorption is
          diminished
   C   will only opacify the gallbladder when the serum bilirubin is
          less than 3 mg/100 ml (51 μmol/1)
   D   demonstrates evidence of cholelithiasis in less than 70 per
          cent of affected patients

298 A **True**   this association tends to distinguish the condition
                   from other causes of jaundice such as hepatitis and
                   neoplasia of the pancreas or bile ducts.

   B **False**   only about 75 per cent of cases of choledocholithiasis
                   produce jaundice.

   C **True**   especially if the common bile duct is dilated, if the
                   gallbladder contains multiple small stones or if the
                   operative cholangiogram demonstrates filling defects
                   within the common bile duct.

   D **True**   though the simpler procedure of choledochotomy and
                   removal of stones is sufficient in the majority of cases,
                   it may be indicated if there is a stenosis of the ampulla
                   of Vater or if residual intrahepatic calculi exist.

299 A **False**   approximately 10 per cent of patients with
                   cholecystitis have stones in the common bile duct.
                   These stones usually originate in the gallbaldder.

   B **True**   this is a classical presentation (Charcot's triad).

   C **False**   the jaundice is typically intermittent and thus
                   distinguishable from the jaundice of a malignant
                   obstruction which is progressive.

   D **True**   the gallbladder is fibrotic and non-distensible due to
                   accompanying chronic cholecystitis. Courvoisier first
                   noted that an obstructive jaundice associated with an
                   enlarged palpable gallbladder is usually due to
                   malignancy. Mucoceles and empyemata of the
                   gallbladder provide an exception to this rule.

300 A **True**   failure of opacification of the biliary tree and
   B **True**   gallbladder is frequently due to cystic duct obstruction
   C **True**   by a gallstone or chronic cholecystitis. Lack of
                   absorption of the oral medium, or failure of the liver to
                   concentrate it when liver function is impaired, may
                   produce this effect.

   D **False**   oral cholecystography is one of the most reliable
                   contrast radiological techniques of the
                   gastrointestinal tract. It will produce evidence of
                   gallbladder disease in more than 90 per cent of
                   affected patients.

301   In severe jaundice diagnostic evidence of an extrahepatic obstruction of the biliary tract may be gained by
  A   intravenous cholangiography
  B   a barium meal
  C   endoscopic retrograde cholangiography
  D   percutaneous transhepatic cholangiography

302   Internal biliary fistulae
  A   most commonly arise as a consequence of cholecystitis
  B   most commonly occur between the gallbladder and the duodenum
  C   can result in intestinal obstruction
  D   are usually accompanied by cholangitis

303   Carcinoma of the gallbladder
  A   is usually a squamous cell neoplasm
  B   is more common in men
  C   is usually associated with gallstones
  D   has a relatively poor prognosis

304   Hypersplenism
  A   results in anaemia, leucopenia and thrombocytopenia
  B   only occurs in the presence of a large spleen
  C   frequently follows liver cirrhosis
  D   may be diagnosed by bone marrow biopsy

301 A **False**   if the serum bilirubin is above 4 to 5 mg/100 ml (68 to 85 μmol/1) no visualisation of the biliary tract will be achieved.
   B **True**   a barium meal will yield information about the head of
   C **True**   the pancreas and the ampullary region but this
   D **True**   indirect and rather unreliable investigation has been replaced by one or other of the following two investigations. Retrograde cannulation of the ampulla allows cholangiography to be achieved directly and is occasionally of great diagnostic value. Percutaneous transhepatic cholangiography may yield valuable information prior to laparotomy if the intrahepatic bile ducts are obstructed and distended.

302 A **True**   by far the commonest cause is an inflamed
   B **True**   gallbladder becoming adherent to a neighbouring
   C **True**   viscus and the contained gallstones eroding into this viscus. More than 75 per cent of these fistulae are between the gallbladder and duodenum. Occasionally the passage of gallstones into the intestinal tract results in intestinal obstruction, usually in the terminal ileum, the narrowest part of the intestinal tract.
   D **False**   though cholangitis may occasionally be a complication, it is rare — many such fistulae close without treatment.

303 A **False**   the majority are adenocarcinomas and are much more
   B **False**   common in females. The incidence is highest in the
   C **True**   elderly and more than 90 per cent of cases are
   D **True**   associated with gallstones. It is widely believed, but not proven, that calculous cholecystitis is an aetiological factor. The symptoms are usually similar in the two conditions. The 5-year survival is less than 5 per cent — the tumour is usually advanced at the time of presentation.

304 A **True**   hypersplenism produces trapping of the formed elements of the blood within the spleen and an abnormally high rate of destruction of red and white blood cells and platelets.
   B **True**   hypersplenism is always the result of a hypertrophied spleen either by inflammatory, infiltrative or congestive processes. Splenectomy usually reverses these changes.
   C **True**   any process which produces portal hypertension may result in hypersplenism.
   D **True**   increased erythropoiesis and an excess of megakaryocytes will be noted.

305   Acute pancreatitis
   A has a higher incidence in alcoholics
   B is commonly associated with the presence of gallstones
   C occurs most commonly in diabetics
   D becomes more severe with each recurring episode.

306   Acute pancreatitis is characterised by
   A a history of gallstones
   B diffuse epigastric pain
   C exaggerated bowel sounds
   D an elevated urinary diastase

307   Chronic pancreatitis
   A is commonly associated with alcoholism
   B is associated with diabetes
   C may be diagnosed by the analysis of pancreatic secretions
   D may be treated by surgical procedures which decompress the
       pancreatic duct.

305 A **True**   the aetiology of this condition is unknown, but biliary
    B **True**   reflux into the pancreatic duct and spasm of the
    C **False** sphincter of Oddi are thought to be important. In
                 Britain about half the patients have co-existing
                 gallstones. Though only a small proportion have
                 stones found in the common bile duct there is
                 evidence that temporary ampullary obstruction by a
                 gallstone that is subsequently discharged into the
                 duodenum is quite common. There is an increased
                 incidence in alcoholics and in the USA this is the most
                 commonly associated condition. It does not occur
                 very commonly in diabetics.
    D **False** it is usual that the first attack is the most severe.
                 Further attacks usually decrease in severity.

306 A **True**   in the United Kingdom gallstones are associated in
                 approximately 40 per cent of cases. In the USA
                 alcoholism is by far the commonest associated factor.
    B **True**   the pain may be slow in onset but often becomes
                 severe, constant and radiating to the back and the left
                 flank.
    C **False** bowel sounds are diminished or absent in severe
                 cases because of the associated paralytic ileus.
    D **True**   the serum amylase is very frequently raised but often
                 for only 24 hours or so. The urinary diastase is
                 similarly elevated but for 1 or 2 days longer. It is thus a
                 more useful diagnostic tool.

307 A **True**   the fundamental cause of this condition is as obscure
                 as that of acute pancreatitis but biliary tract disease
                 and alcoholism are again frequently associated.
    B **True**   chronic epigastric pain radiating to the back, diabetes,
                 steatorrhoea and weight loss combine to form the
                 classical presentation.
    C **True**   diagnosis may be difficult but the enzyme content of
                 the pancreatic secretions secreted in response to
                 hormonal or food stimulation is frequently diminished.
    D **True**   pancreatic duct obstruction is the usual cause of the
                 progression of the disease, thus sphincteroplasty or
                 drainage of the duct into the jejunum may be
                 employed with moderately good results. If gallstones
                 are present cholecystectomy should be performed.

308   Pancreatic pseudocysts
A   are developmental in origin
B   usually arise in the lesser peritoneal sac
C   produce a smooth epigastric mass which moves on
    respiration
D   may be effectively treated by internal drainage

309   The Zollinger-Ellison syndrome
A   is the result of hypergastrinaemia
B   is produced by parietal cell neoplasia
C   includes diarrhoea and malabsorption among its presenting
    features
D   is most effectively treated by total gastrectomy

310   Tumours of the Zollinger-Ellison type
A   may be associated with hyperparathyroidism
B   often produce unusual duodenal ulcers
C   are frequently malignant
D   may be treated medically

308 A **False** there is usually a history of preceding pancreatitis or trauma. They arise following rupture of a pancreatic duct and the subsequent leakage of pancreatic secretions into the retroperitoneal tissues.

    B **True** they are thus commonly related to surrounding organs, the stomach, liver and colon.

    C **False** though a smooth mass can usually be palpated, it does not move on respiration.

    D **True** internal drainage of the cyst into the stomach or small bowel is the preferred treatment providing the cyst is not infected and its wall is well formed. Pancreatic abscesses should be drained externally.

309 A **True** in this syndrome excessive amounts of gastrin are
    B **False** produced by non-beta cell islet tumours of the pancreas. 50 per cent of these tumours are malignant and metastasise to lymph nodes and the liver. The tumours are frequently multiple.

    C **True** there is a very high acid secretion, more than 15 mEq (15 mmol)/hr. It is thought that this high acid secretion inactivates lipase to produce steatorrhoea and diarrhoea.

    D **True** because of the multiplicity of the tumours in the pancreas, surgical removal of single tumours is rarely successful in reducing the gastric hypersecretory state. Removal of the 'target' organ by total gastrectomy is thus preferred.

310 A **True** gastrinomas and hyperparathyroidism are associated in the multiple endocrine abnormality syndrome (Type 1)

    B **True** the commonest presentation is for the patient to demonstrate recurrent duodenal ulceration after apparently adequate therapy or for peptic ulcers to appear in the second and third parts of the duodenum or in the jejunum. The diagnosis is confirmed by finding high levels of serum gastrin.

    C **True** the majority are malignant and multiple tumours are common.

    D **True** after a negative abdominal exploration some authorities are now recommending that cimetidine in larger than normal doses, will control effects of gastrinomas. Whether it can control its rate of growth and spread remains to be seen.

311   Cancer of the pancreas
A   occurs commonly in the head of the pancreas
B   is decreasing in incidence in the Western World
C   is not related to diabetes mellitus
D   is related to cigarette smoking

312   Cancer of the pancreas
A   produces epigastric discomfort
B   produces abdominal pain which is usually relieved by lying down
C   frequently cannot be precisely diagnosed prior to laparotomy
D   is usually treated by radical surgery

311 A **True**   70 per cent of the adenocarcinomas arise in the head
                     of the pancreas.
     B **False**   its incidence has tripled in the last 40 years.
     C **False**   there is an association between pancreatic cancer and
                     diabetes. There is some evidence of an excess
                     incidence in diabetes and, additionally pancreatic
                     cancer is often diagnosed within a year of diabetes
                     appearing in an elderly patient.
     D **False**

312 A **True**   vague abdominal pain and weight loss are the earliest
     B **False**   signs and these often only appear when the cancer is
                     at an advanced stage. Later the pain usually radiates
                     to the back and is worse on lying down. Jaundice
                     frequently complicates cancer of the head of the
                     pancreas.
     C **True**   the barium meal may show effacement of the greater
                     curvature of the stomach or the duodenal loop — but
                     this is a late and inconstant sign. No precise
                     biochemical diagnostic test exists and radioisotope
                     scanning is imprecise. Cytology of pancreatic fluid is
                     yielding good results in some centres. Mesenteric
                     arteriography may demonstrate some tumours but at
                     present laparotomy is the most certain method of
                     diagnosis.
     D **False**   radical surgery can only be undertaken in a small
                     proportion of cases since the majority of patients have
                     such advanced disease that only palliative measures
                     are possible.

15 Genito-urinary tract

313 Haematuria
- **A** at the beginning of micturition is usually indicative of urethral pathology
- **B** at the end of micturition is usually due to bladder neck pathology
- **C** thoughout the urinary stream is typical of renal pathology
- **D** in elderly males is usually related to benign prostatic hypertrophy

314 An intravenous pyelogram
- **A** yields most diagnostic information when performed on a well hydrated patient
- **B** should be preceded by a plain film of the abdomen
- **C** normally shows incomplete filling of the ureter in any one exposure
- **D** should provide evidence of the presence, if any, of lower urinary tract obstruction

315 Wilms' tumours
- **A** metastasise readily to the lungs
- **B** metastasise readily to the bones
- **C** are occasionally bilateral
- **D** have the worst prognosis of all childhood abdominal tumours

313 A **True**   this pattern of haematuria is due to a lesion situated distal to the external sphincter.

B **True**   this pattern of haematuria is caused by pathology in the region of the bladder neck, trigone or posterior urethra.

C **True**   infection, neoplasia and blood dyscrasias should be considered.

D **True**   this is the commonest cause of haematuria in elderly males. The bleeding arises from fragile veins over the urethral surface of the gland.

314 A **False**   better renal concentration is achieved when the patient is slightly dehydrated.

B **True**   this often shows the renal size and the majority of renal and ureteric calculi.

C **True**   peristalsis of the healthy ureter ensures that it is incompletely filled by contrast. If complete filling of the ureter is demonstrated then some degree of ureteric obstruction should be suspected.

D **True**   films should be taken of the bladder after micturition. In the healthy bladder there is an insignificant residue, whereas in bladder neck obstruction there is an increased post-micturition residue.

315 A **True**   this embryonal neoplasm (nephroblastoma) usually presents with an abdominal mass and haematuria. Pulmonary metastases are seen in more than 25 per cent of cases on presentation.

B **False**   in contradistinction to neuroblastomata and adult renal cancers, bone metastases are rare.

C **True**   up to 6 per cent of cases have been shown to have bilateral tumours.

D **False**   aggressive 'triple therapy' with radical excision of the primary tumour and associated lymph nodes, postoperative radiotherapy to the primary site and areas of metastasis together with postoperative actinomycin D or vincristine result in high cure rates (90 per cent where no metastases are present and 40 per cent where lymph node metastases have occurred).

316   **Renal artery stenosis**
  A   is a common cause of hypertension
  B   is most commonly caused by fibro-muscular hyperplasia
  C   can usually be diagnosed on an intravenous pyelogram
  D   should be treated by nephrectomy

317   **In renal transplantation**
  A   a donor kidney may be used from a patient with malignancy
      provided there is no abdominal involvement
  B   ABO compatibility between donor and recipient does not
      have to be considered
  C   satisfactory renal function can be expected with a warm
      ischaemic time of up to 200 minutes
  D   the characteristic signs of acute rejection include pyrexia,
      hypertension and leucocytosis

316 A **False**   this uncommon cause of hypertension usually
presents as an abrupt onset of hypertension in a
middle aged patient. (The practice of screening all
hypertensive patients for the condition by intravenous
pyelography has been unproductive.)

   B **False**   the commonest cause is atheromatous narrowing of
the renal artery.

   C **True**   a slight decrease in renal size, delay in opacification of
the renal pelvis and late hyperconcentration of
contrast medium (due to excessive tubular
reabsorption of water) are all suggestive of the
condition.

   D **False**   careful assessment of the patient's general condition
including the function of the opposite kidney and the
nature of the arterial occlusion lead to surgical
treatment being advised in approximately half of the
younger patients. Usually this is by arterial
reconstruction although nephrectomy is occasionally
necessary.

317 A **False**   patients with malignancy are unsuitable donors, as
are the aged, patients with renal disease or
hypertension. Best results are obtained when the
donor organ is from a living blood relative. The most
satisfactory cadaver donors are young patients dying
of head injuries.

   B **False**   donor and recipient must be ABO compatible;
otherwise, hyperacute rejection may occur within a
few minutes.

   C **False**   maximum renal function is obtained with warm
ischaemic times of under 30 minutes, if this time
exceeds 100 minutes it cannot be expected and the
kidney should not be transplanted. Recently some
success in extending the ischaemic time by tissue
perfusion has been reported.

   D **True**   acute rejection is seen during the first 3 months after
transplantation. Some success has been achieved in
treating such episodes with high doses of steroids and
immunosuppressive drugs.

318　An adenocarcinoma of the kidney
    A　usually occurs in the 35 to 45 age group
    B　usually presents with a urinary infection
    C　is often indistinguishable from a renal cyst radiologically
    D　frequently invades and grows along the renal artery

319　Tumours of the renal pelvis
    A　usually present as a mass in the loin
    B　are possibly due to a urinary carcinogen
    C　resemble those of the bladder in their pathology
    D　are best treated by a partial or total nephrectomy

320　Ureteric calculi
    A　often result from urinary tract infection
    B　frequently cause haematuria
    C　are not usually radio-opaque
    D　producing ureteric colic should be surgically removed

321　Cancer of the penis
    A　is more common in the circumcised
    B　commonly arises from the corona of glans penis
    C　Is usually an adenocarcinoma
    D　Rarely metastasises

318 A **False**   it usually occurs between the age of 50 to 70 years and it is rare before the age of 30.

   B **False**   haematuria, loin pain and a mass are the usual symptoms but they may be preceded by general malaise or the symptoms of a bony metastasis.

   C **True**   the differential diagnosis from the more common condition of renal cysts usually requires further investigations such as selective renal angiography or ultrasound studies.

   D **False**   the renal vein is commonly involved by the tumour growing along it and sometimes reaching the inferior vena cava where it may embolise.

319 A **False**   although on rare occasions the tumour may block the ureter and give rise to hydronephrosis the usual presentation is with haematuria and clot colic.

   B **True**   tumours of the renal pelvis resemble those of the bladder in that they may be due to a urinary carcinogen.

   C **True**   they are carcinomas arising from transitional epithelium.

   D **False**   their spread is by seedlings to ureter and bladder. They are therefore treated by nephrectomy and ureterectomy, the latter being extended to include an adjacent cuff of bladder wall.

320 A **True**   infection, stasis, prolonged immobilisation and generalised metabolic diseases such as gout, hyperparathyroidism and cystinuria may cause urinary calculi.

   B **True**   this may not be overt but urinalysis usually reveals erythrocytes in the urine.

   C **False**   more than 90 per cent of ureteric calculi are radio-opaque. Uric acid calculi are not.

   D **False**   most stones measuring less than 4 mm diameter on X-ray will pass spontaneously.

321 A **False**   it is very much commoner in the uncircumcised and is commonest amongst Social Class V

   B **True**   this is much the commonest site where it may be hidden by the foreskin.

   C **False**   it is a squamous cell carcinoma.

   D **False**   inguinal lymph node metastases are common. Infection of the neoplasm may also produce enlarged regional nodes and care should be taken to distinguish infective from neoplastic lymph node enlargement.

322   Carcinoma of the prostate
   A   is commonly of squamous cell origin
   B   usually originates in the periphery of the gland
   C   usually presents relatively early with lower urinary tract
       symptoms
   D   can be readily diagnosed on rectal examination

323   Carcinoma of the prostate
   A   does not usually metastasise
   B   usually produces an elevated serum acid phosphatase
   C   can be effectively treated by hormones
   D   is most effectively treated by surgery

324   Benign prostatic hypertrophy
   A   is the result of hyperplasia of the fibromuscular capsule of the
       gland
   B   results in diminished power of urination
   C   results in terminal dribbling of urine
   D   often presents with haematuria

322 A **False** adenocarcinoma is by far the most common form
   B **True** particularly in the posterior part of the capsule
   C **False** unfortunately symptoms are not present in the early stages of prostatic cancer. Its peripheral origin ensures that urethral involvement occurs late in the disease.
   D **True** the advanced case demonstrates a nodular diffuse hardness often with fixation to surrouding structures. The early case will present as a solitary hard nodule which must be considered carcinoma until proved otherwise.

323 A **False** metastases are very common and are often blood borne, thus the skeleton, particularly the sacrum and lumbar spine, and the lungs are frequently involved.
   B **True** small tumours and those with a low metabolic activity may be associated with normal values.
   C **True** bilateral orchidectomy or daily stilboestral has been frequently shown to be associated with good 10-year survival rates, regardless of the stage of the disease. However, in some patients the risks of oestrogen therapy (congestive cardiac failure and cerebral and coronary thrombosis) may be higher than the risks of the disease.
   D **False** less than 10 per cent of patients have cancer limited to the gland and radical surgery should only be offered to fit patients with a relatively long life expectancy.

324 A **False** senile prostatic hyperplasia follows proliferation of the central periurethral glandular tissue. A lobular growth pattern usually involves either the median lobe beneath the bladder trigone or the lateral lobes. The peripheral capsule of the gland is displaced and compressed by this process.
   B **True** as the hyperplasia develops the prostatic urethra
   C **True** narrows and elongates and a mechanical obstruction
   D **True** to micturition develops. The force and size of the stream decreases. Frequency and terminal dribbling often indicate an increased residual urine and dysuria resulting from infection is common. Haematuria occurs quite commonly and results from damage to engorged urethral veins during micturition.

325 **Benign prostatic hypertrophy**
   A   can readily be assessed on rectal examination
   B   can be effectively treated with hormones
   C   is most effectively treated by surgery
   D   is a premalignant condition

326 **Acute prostatitis**
   A   is most commonly due to coliform organisms
   B   often presents as an ache in the perineum
   C   may be diagnosed by rectal examination
   D   requires bladder catheterisation as part of the treatment

327 **Urethral strictures**
   A   rarely cause dysuria
   B   are confined to the membranous urethra
   C   are frequently traumatic
   D   produce perineal abscesses

328 **Bladder cancer**
   A   may follow exposure to beta-naphthylamine
   B   is more common in heavy smokers
   C   is more common in females
   D   is frequently associated with bladder schistosomiasis

325 A **False**   rectal assessment of prostate size is not reliable for the median lobe is impalpable. (The degree of prostatic hypertrophy is not related to the amount of urinary obstruction. Small glands may produce obstruction and large glands none.)

     B **False**   hormonal therapy has not yet proved satisfactory.

     C **True**   though the general condition of the patient and the extent of his disability must always be considered.

     D **False**   there is no firm evidence relating benign hyperplasia with neoplasia of the gland.

326 A **True**   *Escherichia coli* is the commonest organism isolated. Acute gonococcal prostatitis may also occur.

     B **True**   this is a common symptom together with dysuria, urgency and frequency. Fever and rigors are often present.

     C **True**   the prostate is diffusely enlarged and very tender.

     D **False**   instrumentation of the lower urinary tract should be avoided, unless urinary retention is present, for bacteraemic shock may follow. Broad spectrum antibiotics should be prescribed for at least 2 weeks.

327 A **False**   difficulty in micturition is common and infections of the urinary tract are commonly associated.

     B **False**   strictures of the external meatus may follow chronic

     C **False**   balanitis; congenital strictures may occur because of posterior urethral valves; gonorrhea and bilharziasis can produce strictures anywhere along the length of the urethra, and traumatic strictures usually affect the bulbous or membranous parts of the urethra.

     D **True**   extravasation of infected urine frequently causes. peno-scrotal abscesses and when these discharge to the skin urinary fistulae will follow.

328 A **True**   industrial and laboratory use of this chemical is now very strictly controlled.

     B **True**   although a urinary carcinogen has not yet been isolated in these patients.

     C **False**   it is 3 to 4 times commoner in males and occurs mainly in the sixth and seventh decades.

     D **True**   schistosoma haematobium is thought to predispose to bladder cancer. There is a high incidence of bladder cancer in regions where schistosomiasis is endemic.

329   Bladder cancers
   A   are usually adenocarcinomas
   B   are usually ulcerating
   C   usually present with suprapubic pain radiating to the
       perineum
   D   are usually diagnosed on excretory pyelography

330   Undescended testes
   A   are often associated with inguinal herniae
   B   usually descend at puberty
   C   can usually be made to descend by the examiner with warm
       hands
   D   should be treated by orchidopexy at puberty

329 A **False**   these are rare. The commonest neoplasm is a
    B **False**   transitional cell carcinoma and these usually from
                  sessile tumours which only occasionally ulcerate.
    C **False**   this is a sign of advanced and incurable disease. The
                  commonest presenting sign is of painless intermittent
                  haematuria which may later become associated with
                  symptoms of cystitis and strangury (pain at the end of
                  micturition).
    D **False**   the intravenous pyelogram frequently shows no
                  disturbance of renal function. Only large bladder
                  cancers will be revealed on the cystogram.
                  Cystoscopy is the most reliable method of diagnosis
                  and should be performed in all patients suspected of
                  the disease.

330 A **True**   this relatively common abnormality (which occurs in 2
                  to 4 per cent of male children) is usually associated
                  with a patent processus vaginalis and an inguinal
                  hernia.
    B **False**   this is rare, and usually means that the original
                  diagnosis should have been that of a retractile testis.
    C **False**   undescended testes cannot be brought below the
                  neck of the scrotum. Those that can be encouraged
                  into the scrotum are merely retractile and not
                  pathological.
    D **False**   surgical replacement of the testis into the scrotum as
                  soon as is feasible, say by the age of 3 years, ensures
                  normal spermatogenesis and may decrease the
                  higher incidence of neoplasia that occurs in
                  abdominal testes.

331   Unilateral undescended testes are associated with
   A   infertility
   B   malignancy
   C   torsion
   D   drainage by trauma

332   The spermatic cord contains
   A   the inferior epigastric vein
   B   the deep circumflex iliac artery
   C   the pudendal nerve
   D   the subcostal nerve

333   Torsion of the spermatic cord
   A   often presents with vomiting and lower abdominal pain
   B   often produces gangrene of the testis
   C   may initially be treated effectively by non-surgical means
   D   always requires surgical treatment

334   Seminomas of the testis
   A   most commonly occur before the age of 40
   B   are usually sensitive to radiotherapy
   C   rarely metastasise via the blood stream
   D   generally carry a poor prognosis

331 A **False**   bilateral undescent of the testis is associated with infertility
     B **True**   the risk of malignancy is some 30–40 times greater. Orchidopexy before the age of 5 years may be effective in reducing this risk.
     C **True**   because it is often lying loosely in a hernial sac the undescended testis frequently undergoes torsion. Diagnosis is delayed unless the scrotum is examined.
     D **True**   the testis position, often overlying the pubic tubercle increases its risk of drainage by trauma.

332 A **False**   the spermatic cord is invested with external and
     B **False**   internal spermatic fascia together with the cremaster
     C **False**   muscle. It contains testicular vessels, the vas
     D **False**   deferens, the ilio-inguinal nerve and sympathetic nerve fibres. A patent processus vaginalis is present in those patients with an indirect inguinal hernia.

333 A **True**   together with the sudden onset of severe testicular pain.
     B **True**   this is almost inevitable unless the torsion is corrected within 12 hours.
     C **True**   manual correction, by rotating the testis in the direction which is the least painful is often successful in releasing the torsion.
     D **True**   fixation of the abnormally mobile testis (and its opposite number) is always indicated even if initial relief has been obtained by non-surgical means.

334 A **True**   though they may occur at any age more than 80 per cent occur before the age of 40.
     B **True**   the majority are radiosensitive and, since blood borne
     C **True**   metastases are less common, surgical removal of the
     D **False**   affected testis combined with radio-therapy to the iliac and para-aortic nodes produce 5-year survival rates of up to 90 per cent. Teratomas of the testis are less radio-sensitive, metastasise more frequently via the blood stream and have a much worse prognosis.

335   A teratoma of the testis
A   may contain ectodermal or endodermal but not mesodermal cells
B   has a 5-year survival of up to 80 per cent in the teratoma differentiated (TD) variety
C   may be diagnosed by the Aschheim-Zondek pregnancy test
D   should only be treated by radiotherapy in incurable cases

336   Hypospadias
A   is the result of failure of scrotal development
B   results in the abnormal urethra opening into the dorsum of the penis
C   is associated with chordee
D   is associated with maldescent of the testis

335 A **False**   these tumours arise from the totipotent cells of the rete testis and may be of any germ layer, one form being usually predominant.

B **True**   survival figures vary with the histological type, TD

C **True**   having the best prognosis while the malignant

D **False**   teratoma trophoblastic, MTT (which may have a positive pregnancy test) has an extremely poor prognosis. The introduction of routine prophylactic radiotherapy to the para-aortic nodes and combination chemotherapy with a cis-platinum vinblastine and bleomycin has, with these tumours as well as the seminoma, markedly improved survival figures.

336 A **False**   it is the result of incomplete development of the anterior urethra.

B **False**   in hypospadias the urethra opens onto the ventral aspect of the glans or penile shaft.

C **True**   in severe cases the fibrous remnant of the undeveloped urethra gives an abnormal downward curvature to the penis.

D **True**   this is rare but the resulting state of the external genitalia may produce a state of intersex.

56 % on 20/2/91
73 % on 23/3/91
81 % on 10/4/91

16 Lymphatic and vascular systems

337 The protein content of the lymph
- **A** from the liver is over 5 g/100 ml (50 g/l)
- **B** from the periphery is 2 g/100 ml (20 g/l)
- **C** from the gastrointestinal tract is 3 to 5 g/100 ml (30 to 50 g/l)
- **D** in the thoracic duct is 8 g/100 ml (80 g/l)

338 The lymphatic vessels
- **A** of most tissues bear a direct numerical relation to the vascular capillaries
- **B** of the pyloric antrum pass directly to the lymphatic duct without traversing any lymph nodes
- **C** drain 50 per cent of the arterial capillary filtrate
- **D** are almost totally responsible for the reabsorption of protein from the interstitial fluid

339 The lymphatic vessels draining
- **A** the stomach pass with the veins to the caval plexuses
- **B** the tip of the tongue pass to the submental nodes
- **C** the lower anal canal pass to the inguinal nodes
- **D** the upper extremity differ from that of the lower extremity in that they follow the veins

340 The lymph nodes
- **A** of the axilla number up to 20
- **B** of the parotid group drain the inner ear and external auditory meatus
- **C** of the left supraclavicular fossa are commonly implicated in gastrointestinal malignancy
- **D** are responsible for the production of plasma cells

337 A **True**
    B **True**
    C **True**
    D **False**   since it is a mixture of lymph from all sources, its
                   protein content is 3 to 5 g/100 ml (30 to 50 g/l).

338 A **True**   rare exceptions being the central nervous system and
                   the spleen which contain no lymphatic capillaries
    B **False**   this is only true of the lymph vessels from the thyroid,
                   oesophagus, heart and adrenals, the remainder
                   traverse at least one and sometimes as many as 10
                   lymph nodes.
    C **False**   total lymph production is about 120 ml/hour (about 10
                   per cent of the capillary filtrate).
    D **True**   only a small proportion of filtered protein diffuses
                   back to the venous capillaries.

339 A **False** the gastric lymph vessels accompany the arteries (the
                   regional nodes are named after them) before passing
                   to the coeliac and superior mesenteric pre-aortic
                   nodes.
    B **True**   the lateral aspect drains to submandibular nodes and
                   the posterior third to retropharyngeal nodes.
    C **True**   but those of the upper anal canal pass to the inferior
                   mesenteric nodes. This is an important factor in
                   deciding the surgical approach to neoplasms of the
                   anal canal.
    D **False**   the lymphatics of both upper and lower limbs follow
                   the veins.

340 A **False** as many as 30 to 60 may be present, receiving the
                   dermal lymphatics from the trunk and arm and also
                   the majority of the breast tissue lymphatics.
    B **True**   the lymphatics draining the face also pass to this
                   group. In malignant lesions of the face with nodal
                   involvement a superficial parotidectomy may be
                   necessary as the nodes are embedded in the gland.
    C **True**   this was observed by Virchow who was the first to link
                   the lymphatic system with the spread of malignant
                   disease.
    D **True**   these are involved in the production of humoral
                   antibodies.

341   **A cystic hygroma**
  A   is a lymphangioma
  B   occurs most commonly in the second year of life
  C   is usually situated in the posterior mediastinum
  D   usually regresses at puberty

342   **Lymphoedema tarda**
  A   is a late complication of venous thrombosis
  B   should be treated by varicose vein surgery
  C   can be improved by postural drainge
  D   should be treated with prophylactic antibiotics

343   **Secondary lymphoedema**
  A   may be caused by *Wuchereria bancrofti*
  B   of the arm in post-mastectomy patients undergoes
      lymphosarcomatous changes in 10 per cent of patients
  C   is characterised by an increased number of lymphatics
  D   is characterised by dermal backflow

344   **The treatment of lymphangitis in a limb should include**
  A   active mobilisation to allow the muscle pump to maintain
      lymph flow
  B   incision of any associated inflamed areas
  C   the use of an appropriate antibiotic
  D   lymphangiography

341 A **True** which is usually congenital in origin.
    B **False** the majority occur in the first year. 90 per cent have occurred before the end of the second year.
    C **False** it is usually situated in the neck.
    D **False** it may grow considerably during early childhood. Regression is very uncommon. Surgical cure is difficult but is indicated occasionally for cosmetic reasons or to relieve tracheal compression.

342 A **False** it is a primary lymphoedema of late onset.
    B **False** venous surgery should be avoided since any lymphatics that are present follow the veins and may be damaged.
    C **True** together with compression bandaging of the legs when the patient is ambulant.
    D **False** antibiotic therapy in lymphoedema is necessary when these are frequently recurring attacks of cellulitis.

343 A **True** the filarial larvae are transmitted by mosquitos. The adult worm lives primarily in the lymphatic vessels and nodes, causing lymphatic obstruction.
    B **False** this rare malignancy occurs in less than 0.5 per cent of such patients.
    C **False** the number of lymphatics is not increased but they are dilated.
    D **True** this is usually revealed by contrast radiology and demonstrates stasis and distension in the skin lymphatics.

344 A **False** rest and elevation reduces the lymph flow and help to localise infection.
    B **False** only if an abscess is present is incision indicated.
    C **True** lymphangitis indicates a failure of localisation of the infection and thus antibiotics should be used.
    D **False** this investigation has no place in the management of lymphangitis.

345   **Acute arterial occlusion**
   A   should be treated conservatively if the site of the occlusion is above the inguinal ligament
   B   demands the urgent use of vasodilator drugs
   C   of a limb is usually painless due to the anoxic damage produced in the peripheral nerves
   D   may produce irreversible muscle necrosis after 6 hours

346   **In chronic arterial occlusion of the lower limbs**
   A   buttock claudication is suggestive of arterial occlusion above the inguinal ligament
   B   skin ulceration most commonly occurs along the medial border of the foot
   C   which is severe, there may be venous 'guttering' on elevation of the legs
   D   there is usually an associated peripheral neuropathy

347   **Chronic arterial occlusion of the lower limb results in**
   A   muscle atrophy
   B   brittle nails
   C   ischaemic nerve pain
   D   paradoxical warmth in the foot

345 A **False**   gangrene of the lower limbs frequently follows
untreated saddle emboli and iliac vessel occlusion.
Urgent surgical removal of the clot is thus indicated in
the majority of patients.

B **False**   there are no pharmacological agents available which
can improve on the vasodilatation that has already
occurred in the ischaemic area.

C **False**   the pain is immediate and severe and worsens as
muscle necrosis develops.

D **True**   the onset of this condition which soon becomes
irreversible is indicated by the development of
tenderness and spasm in the muscles together with
muscle swelling. In such cases it may be necessary to
decompress the muscular compartment by
fasciotomy in addition to relieving the arterial
obstruction.

346 A **True**   it is particularly common in internal iliac artery
occlusion and therefore with severe disease of the
common iliac arteries or the aorta.

B **False**   the commonest sites of skin ulceration are of the toes
and in the interdigital clefts. Trauma frequently results
in the heel or the lateral border of the foot becoming
ulcerated.

C **True**   this, together with pallor on elevation and redness on
dependency indicate a very inadequate arterial supply
which is neither sufficient to produce venous filling
nor to prevent anoxic vasodilation of the skin vessels.

D **False**   this is uncommon in uncomplicated chronic arterial
obstruction. It does occur in diabetic patients with
arterial disease and contributes to the high incidence
of foot ulceration in these patients.

347 A **True**   muscle atrophy is common and most marked when
B **True**   the leg vessels are occluded. Absence of hair and slow
growing brittle nails are common.

C **True**   rest pain, initially felt at night and relieved by foot
dependency, is due to nerve ischaemia.

D **False**   the limb is cold and feels cold.

348   Abdominal aortic aneurysms
   A arise from an atheromatous vessel in approximately 50 per
        cent of cases
   B characteristically produce epigastric pain
   C are associated with duodenal ulceration
   D which are asymptomatic are relatively benign conditions and
        should not usually be resected

349   Raynaud's disease
   A is caused by an abnormal sensitivity of skin vessels to cold
   B is marked by a characteristic pallor of the hands after cold
        stimulation followed by blue and then red colour changes
   C may be associated with scleroderma
   D is permanently relieved by sympathectomy in the vast
        majority of cases.

350   Common sites for atheromatous arterial aneurysms are
   A the femoral artery
   B the middle cerebral artery
   C the abdominal aorta
   D intrarenal

348 A **False**   over 95 per cent of these aneurysms are
                    atheromatous, the remainder are syphilitic, traumatic
                    or mycotic in origin.

   B **False**   the majority of aortic aneurysms are painless.
                    However, when enlargement does occur, pain is felt in
                    the flanks or in the back.

   C **True**   there is an unexplained increase of duodenal
                    ulceration in patients with aortic aneurysms and
                    rupture may occur into the duodenum.

   D **False**   every patient with an aortic aneurysm, whether
                    asymptomatic or not, is at risk of rupture, particularly
                    when the aneurysm is larger than 6 cm or is tender.
                    Only in relatively small aneurysms and in very aged or
                    unfit patients is conservative management indicated.

349 A **True**   the disease has an unknown aetiology and is usually
                    seen only in temperate zones. It is most common in
                    young women appearing in the second and third
                    decades.

   B **True**   these changes are produced by intense and abnormal
                    vasoconstriction which follows cold exposure and
                    then after a period of several minutes' rewarming, an
                    anoxic vasodilation of the skin vessels occurs. There is
                    an initial sluggish and then a more rapid blood flow
                    through the dilated and anoxic skin vessels

   C **False**   collagen diseases, certain haematological disorders,
                    occupational use of vibrating tools and sundry other
                    unrelated diseases may be associated with Raynaud's
                    phenomenon (see B above). Raynaud's disease
                    however is the name given to the idiopathic disease
                    defined in A.

   D **False**   less than three-quarters of the patients with
                    Raynaud's disease are relieved by sympathectomy
                    and of these in only half is the relief permanent.

350 A **True**   these are often bilateral and occur in association with
                    aortic aneurysms.

   B **False**   these are congenital and often produce symptoms
                    before atheromatous changes have occurred, ie.
                    between 20 and 30 years of age.

   C **True**   this is the commonest site. The majority of aortic
                    aneurysms lie below the renal vessels.

   D **False**   when aneurysms occur intrarenally they are usually
                    mycotic (i.e. infective in origin) and multiple.

351   A dissecting aneurysm of the aorta
  A usually starts around the aortic arch
  B is so-called because of the extensive mediastinal destruction
     it produces when it ruptures
  C is associated with pregnancy
  D is a feature of Marfan's syndrome

352   Thromboangitis obliterans
  A was originally described by a Japanese opthalmologist
  B classically involves the branches of the aortic arch
  C is a panarteritis
  D is seen most frequently in young women

353   Varicose veins
  A are common throughout the world
  B are frequently congenital
  C are the commonest cause of venous ulceration
  D are associated with an increased risk of pulmonary
     embolism

354   Commonly used sclerosants for varicose vein injection are
  A 3 per cent sodium tetradecyl sulphate
  B thrombin
  C ethanolamine
  D 5 per cent phenol in almond oil

351 A **True**   the commonest site of origin is just proximal or distal to the origin of the left subclavian artery.
   B **False**   the dissection occurs in the arterial wall and is subintimal. When rupture occurs it is usually retrogradely into the pericardium or distally close to the aortic bifurcation. The effects of an extensive dissection are due to aortic rupture or occlusion aortic branches.
   C **True**   there appears to be an increased incidence in young pregnant women.
   D **True**   this is probably related to defective ground substance and decreased strength in the connective tissue of the arterial wall.

352 A **False**   it was first described by Buerger in 1909.
   B **False**   it characteristically involves medium size arteries of the extremities such as the anterior and posterior tibial, radial and ulnar vessels.
   C **False**   histologically the major effects are found in the intima of the arteries and veins. It is not clear whether these are hypersensitivity phenomena or whether they are just the simple effects of thrombosis in a patient whose blood is 'hypercoagulable'.
   D **False**   thromboangitis obliterans is almost exclusively a disease in males. Cigarette smoking may have a part to play in the aetiology. (All statements in this question are true of Takayasu's disease — a very rare arteritis.)

353 A **False**   they are rare in developing countries.
   B **False**   all are acquired, usually in adulthood. They are commoner in multiparous women but the reasons for this are not known with certainty.
   C **False**   varicose veins alone are a very rare cause of venous ulceration. This almost always follows deep venous thrombosis and its post phlebitic sequelae.
   D **False**   though superficial phlebitis and painful patches of thrombosis are commonly associated these rarely extend into the deep venous system and are not normally a source of pulmonary emboli.

354 A **True**   this detergent compound is used extensively in the technique of compression sclerotherapy for varicose veins.
   B **False**   this could be lethal, giving rise to systemic coagulation effects.
   C **True**   it is a less powerful sclerosant than A.
   D **False**   this solution is used for paravenous injection of haemorrhoids.

355   **In deep venous thrombosis of the lower limb**
    A one of the most common sites of origin is the short saphenous vein
    B one of the common sites of origin is in the iliofemoral segment
    C the diagnosis can usually be made by clinical examination
    D tender swollen thrombosed veins are usually palpable

356   **The incidence of postoperative venous thrombosis can be reduced**
    A by raising the foot of the operating table during surgery
    B by passive calf contractions during an operation
    C by the intravenous administration of 500 ml of low molecular weight Dextran during operation and on the first two postoperative days
    D by the prophylactic use of subcutaneous heparin

357   **Venous ulcers of the lower limb**
    A are usually the result of long-standing varicose veins
    B commonly follow deep venous thrombosis
    C most commonly occur below the medial malleolus
    D will usually heal when firm bandaging is applied

355 A **False** in the lower leg the soleal plexus is the usual site of origin of venous thrombosis.
   B **True** iliofemoral thrombosis commonly follows hip or pelvic surgery and may also extend from the calf veins.
   C **False** there is almost no correlation between signs in the lower leg and the presence of deep vein thrombosis for many thrombi are non-occlusive and produce no ankle swelling or calf tenderness.
   D **False** these are the signs of superficial thrombophlebitis which is not usually related to deep vein thrombosis or associated with the risk of embolism.

356 A **False** this is not of proven value.
   B **True** this reduces venous stasis.
   C **True** this is an effective prophylactic measure and acts by reducing blood viscosity and platelet aggregation.
   D **True** the administration of low doses of heparin in the preoperative and early postoperative period is effective in reducing the incidence of postoperative thrombosis.

357 A **False** uncomplicated varicose veins even if present for many years do not usually produce ulcers, and when they do they are small and heal quickly.
   B **True** 'venous' ulcers are nearly all postphlebitic in origin.
   C **False** the characteristic site is on the medial side of the ankle just above the malleolus.
   D **True** bandaging provides continuous firm compression, preventing oedema and overcoming the increased pressure in the superficial veins of the postphlebitic limb.

17 Fractures and dislocations

358 **A fracture is said to be**
- **A** closed if an overlying skin laceration has been sutured
- **B** comminuted if there has been associated damage to adjacent nerves or vessels
- **C** a fatigue fracture if it occurs through a diseased bone
- **D** pathological if it occurs through a bony metastasis

359 **In a healing fracture**
- **A** the haematoma is initially invaded by osteoblasts
- **B** the tissue formed by the invading osteoblasts is termed osteoid
- **C** calcium salts are laid down in the osteoid tissue
- **D** the final stage of repair is the remodelling of the callus

360 **Non-union is often seen in**
- **A** fractures of the 4th metatarsal
- **B** fractures of the neck of the femur
- **C** fractures of the condyle of the mandible
- **D** Colles' fractures

358 A **False**   a closed fracture does not communicate with the
exterior through a laceration or abrasion of the
overlying skin or mucous membrane. Any fracture
with an associated wound of the overlying skin or
mucosa is said to be an open or compound fracture.

   B **False**   comminuted means that more than 2 fragments of
bone are present. When there is a single fracture line,
the fracture is described as simple, but if the broken
ends are compressed into each other, the fracture is
then said to be impacted.

   C **False**   a fatigue fracture occurs in areas which undergo
repeated stress, an example being the 'march'
fracture of the 4th metatarsal which is usually
sustained by healthy adults after an unaccustomed
long walk.

   D **True**   the term includes fractures through any diseased area
of bone. Other examples include osteoporosis,
osteogenesis imperfecta and Paget's disease.

359 A **False**   the haematoma is initially invaded by capillaries and
fibroblasts. Calcium salts pass into solution in the
acidic environment.

   B **True**   osteoblasts invade the healing wound at 10 to 14
days, the pH progressively becoming more alkaline.
During this time the concentration of alkaline
phosphatase in the wound tissues increases.

   C **True**   this forms callus. The amount formed is to some
extent related to the amount of stress on the fracture
site, thus a fractured femur forms proportionately
much more callus than a fractured metacarpal.

   D **True**   the trabecular architecture of the bone becomes re-
established and excess callus is then reabsorbed.

360 A **False**   classical sites of non-union of fractures are the
   B **True**   scaphoid, talus and the neck of the femur. All the
   C **False**   areas involved are relatively avascular. Delayed union
   D **False**   and non-union are more common in the aged, in
those fractures with associated infection, with
inadequate fixation and when the bony ends are
separated by excessive traction or by the interposition
of soft tissues.

361   Dislocation of the sternoclavicular joint
  A   is usually caused by a fall on the outstretched hand
  B   displaces the clavicle upwards and medially
  C   is usually treated by internal fixation
  D   never causes any compression of the trachea or great vessels
      in the neck

362   Fractures of the clavicle
  A   are usually of the greenstick variety in children under the age
      of 10 years
  B   are usually the result of direct violence
  C   can be recognised by the abnormal elevation of the distal
      fragment
  D   are usually treated by internal fixation

363   In fractures of the surgical neck of the humerus
  A   the lesion is usually due to indirect violence
  B   the fragments are usually impacted
  C   the proximal fragment is usually internally rotated
  D   the distal fragment is usually adducted

361 A **True**   this causes the medial end of the clavicle to rise anteriorly over the sternum.

B **True**   the weight of the arm and the pectoral muscles pull it medially while sternomastoid elevates the medial end of the clavicle.

C **True**   reduction of both anterior and posterior dislocations can be achieved by bracing the shoulders. The attachments of the articular disc which give much of the strength to the joint will have been weakened and dislocation will re-occur unless some form of fixation is undertaken.

D **False**   posterior dislocations may cause the medial end of the clavicle to impinge on the trachea and the great vessels in the neck. Operative reduction is then an urgent necessity.

362 A **True**   thus displacement is minimal and treatment is usually only symptomatic.

B **False**   this fracture is usually due to falls on the outstretched palm. Direct trauma to the outer end usually leads to anterior buckling and injuries to the underlying subclavian vessels and brachial plexus are thus extremely uncommon.

C **False**   the proximal fragment is elevated by the sternomastoid but the distal fragment is depressed by the effect of gravity on the shoulder and arm

D **False**   a figure-of-eight bandage provides some symptomatic relief and support. In most patients the fracture heals without internal fixation. The slight deformity presents few problems.

363 A **True**   the most frequent cause being a fall on the outstretched hand.

B **True**   although the fracture is frequently comminuted, the bone in this region is very cancellous and impacts easily.

C **False**   the rotator cuff muscles are both internal and external rotators of the shoulder. Supinator acts on the proximal fragment producing abduction.

D **True**   the overall displacement is not usually extensive and is accepted. Early mobilisation is encouraged.

364   In a fracture of the distal third of the shaft of the humerus

    A the distal fragment is usually posteriorly angulated by the action of biceps

    B the radial nerve is frequently damaged

    C delayed radial nerve palsy is usually due to oedema

    D late onset of radial nerve palsy is usually due the involvement of the nerve with callus

365   A supracondylar fracture of the humerus

    A is a fracture commonly seen in young adults

    B is particularly subject to the complication of ischaemic muscle contracture

    C is held in the position of reduction by the tendon of brachioradialis

    D when properly reduced has the index finger pointing approximately to the tip of the shoulder of the same side

366   A transverse fracture of the scaphoid is

    A prone to infection

    B usually seen in young men

    C prone to avascular necrosis

    D usually seen on an early scaphoid X-ray

364 A **False**   the elbow is usually held flexed, relaxing biceps, and any angulation is then anterior due to triceps contraction. In proximal fractures of the shaft of the humerus deltoid and pectoralis major muscles both act on the proximal fragment to produce considerable angulation.

B **True**   the radial nerve lies close to the bone in the radial groove and can thus be easily damaged with fracture at this site.

C **False**   if a delayed radial nerve palsy appears, it is almost certainly due to movement and trauma from a sharp fracture surface.

D **True**   if this is the case, then operative treatment and neurolysis (removal of the nerve from the proximity of the healing fracture) may be necessary.

365 A **False**   this is usually a fracture of childhood; and frequently follows a fall on the outstretched hand with the elbow flexed.

B **True**   the brachial artery is frequently traumatised in this lesion and may be lacerated or put into spasm. When this occurs the muscles of the forearm may undergo ischaemic necrosis and contracture.

C **False**   the triceps muscle posteriorly and the brachialis muscle anteriorly are the closest and most powerful relations of this part of the humerus and they have a splinting effect on the reduced fracture.

D **True**   and reduction is keyed by traction on the distal fragment followed by flexion at the elbow. Care must be taken at all times to ensure that the radial pulse is present. It is essential to cut out a window in the plaster at the wrist so that the radial artery can be frequently checked.

366 A **False**   it is rarely compound so infection is not a problem.

B **True**   this injury is sustained by falling on the outstretched hand. In older patients this same injury produces a Colles' fracture.

C **True**   prolonged immobilisation minimises the risk of avascular necrosis and non-union. For this reason plasters are worn until radiological healing is present.

D **False**   fractures of the scaphoid are often not seen on the earliest X-rays and the diagnosis must be made clinically (a painful wrist with tenderness in the anatomical snuff box). Reduction is best achieved with the wrist flexed. Repeat X-rays taken 2 weeks after the injury may then demonstrate some local reabsorption of bone around the fracture and thus render it more obvious.

367   In a Colles' fracture the distal radial fragment
  A   is dorsally angulated on the proximal radius
  B   is usually torn from the intra-articular triangular disc
  C   is deviated to the ulnar side
  D   is usually impacted

368   In a Monteggia fracture dislocation
  A   the dislocation of the distal radio-ulnar joint brings the ulnar styloid process anterior to the capitulum
  B   the radial fracture is usually at the junction of the middle and distal thirds
  C   internal fixation is usually required in the adult
  D   the causative injury is often a blow on the extensor surface of the forearm with the elbow flexed

369   Dislocations of the shoulder joint
  A   most commonly occur in middle age
  B   usually occur when the arm is in the abducted position
  C   usually have the head of the humerus situated behind the glenoid fossa
  D   are often recurrent in the young

370   Fractures of the maxilla
  A   cannot usually be demonstrated radiologically for 48 hours
  B   are often accompanied by numbness over the upper lip
  C   are often accompanied by diplopia
  D   rarely require surgical intervention

367 A **True**   it is also dorsally displaced to produce the typical 'dinner fork' abnormality
    B **False**   the ulna styloid (to which the disc is also attached) is often avulsed but the intra-articular disc of fibrocartilage is far too strong to be torn.
    C **False**   the distal radial fragment is always radially deviated.
    D **True**   therefore reduction of a Colles' fracture should include traction (to overcome impaction), flexion (to overcome dorsal angulation) and ulnar deviation (to overcome radial deviation)

368 A **False**   the dislocation is of the head of the radius from the superior radio-ulnar joint.
    B **False**   the radius is not fractured. The fracture is in the shaft of the ulna at the junction of the proximal and middle thirds.
    C **True**   though in a child the reduction is generally stable.
    D **True**   though it is probably more frequently produced by a fall on the outstretched hand.

369 A **False**   they are commonest in young adults who indulge in athletic pursuits.
    B **True**   the shoulder joint is at its most unstable in this position and may dislocate with a trivial blow.
    C **False**   the head of the humerus is usually displaced anteriorly.
    D **True**   dislocation of the shoulder joint tends to produce laxity in the capsule of the joint and the joint is subsequently less stable.

370 A **False**   if suitable views are taken the fracture lines will be seen immediately and there will be opacity of the appropriate maxillary sinus.
    B **True**   the infraorbital nerve is usually damaged as the fracture line typically passes through the infraorbital canal.
    C **True**   the fracture may involve the bony attachments of the suspensory ligament of the eye.
    D **False**   some form of fixation is usually necessary to avoid persistent diplopia, limitation of jaw movement and cosmetic deformity.

371   In pelvic fractures
   A   avulsion injuries are usually treated by early mobilisation
   B   undisplaced lesions of the ischial or pubic rami are usually
         treated by early mobilisation
   C   extraperitoneal urinary extravasation may be due to damage
         either to the membraneous urethra or to the base of the
         bladder
   D   which are unstable, one half of the pelvis is displaced
         proximally by the flank muscles. Reduction may need 40 to 50
         lb (18 to 23kg) of traction.

372   Intracapsular fractures of the upper end of the femur are usually
   A   accompanied by shortening of the leg
   B   accompanied by external rotation of the leg
   C   accompanied by adduction of the leg
   D   treated by internal fixation

373   Extracapsular fractures of the upper end of the femur are usually
   A   subtrochanteric in position
   B   subject to avascular necrosis of the head of the femur
   C   accompanied by internal rotation of the leg
   D   treated by internal fixation

371 A **True**   these injuries affect the anterior superior and inferior iliac spines and are the result of violent muscle contractions. They do not effect the stability of the pelvis and thus do not require prolonged immobilisation.

B **True**   these injuries are usually due to direct trauma. The stability of the pelvis is not markedly affected and weight bearing can be resumed once the initial pain has subsided.

C **True**   rupture of the puboprostatic ligament may be associated with tearing of the prostate from the membranous urethra. Bony fragments of the fractured pubis may pierce the bladder.

D **True**   in addition, severe pelvic fractures are accompanied by extensive haemorrhage (often concealed), shock and possible bladder and rectal injuries.

372 A **True**   this is the result of the longitudinal pull of the hamstring, rectus femoris and iliopsoas muscles.

B **True**   this is due to the action of iliopsoas acting distal to the fracture.

C **False**   adductor and abductor muscles are both attached to the distal shaft and their actions are thus counterbalanced.

D **True**   this reduces the incidence of avascular necrosis and subsequent non-union. Internal fixation also speeds up mobilisation in these patients who are commonly quite elderly. Very occasionally undisplaced impacted fractures are treated non-surgically.

373 A **False**   the fracture most commonly lies between the greater and lesser trochanters, i.e. is an intertrochanteric fracture.

B **False**   in this type of fracture healing is usually uneventful. The major part of the blood supply to the head of the femur comes through capsular vessels which are usually undamaged in extracapsular fractures.

C **False**   these fractures show shortening and external rotation as in the intracapsular variety. In addition adduction of the leg is present as the adductor muscles act on the distal fragment whithout the opposition of the glutei which remain attached to the proximal fragment.

D **True**   the most commonly used prostheses include a long plate which is screwed onto the upper femoral shaft and a pin which is inserted into the proximal fragment.

374   In fractures of the mid-shaft of the femur
    A the proximal fragment is usually flexed
    B the proximal fragment is usually abducted
    C the distal fragment is usually adducted
    D the common femoral vessels are usually damaged

375   In fractures of the patella
    A comminution is usual when the fracture has been caused by indirect violence
    B a transverse fracture without displacement is usually treated by a plaster cylinder with no direct surgical intervention
    C a comminuted fracture is best treated by patella excision and replacement by a prosthesis
    D weight bearing should be avoided for the first week

376   In fractures of the middle third of the tibia and fibula
    A delayed union is common
    B indirect violence usually results in a spiral or oblique fracture line
    C shortening and anterior angulation of the tibia are common
    D comminuted fractures are usually treated by early plating of the tibia

377   In injuries of the ankle joint
    A eversion injuries are the most commonly encountered
    B inversion injuries are usually accompanied by a tear of the deltoid ligament
    C there is frequently associated posterior tibial nerve damage
    D the joint is rendered unstable by rupture of the inferior tibio-fibular ligament

374 A **True**   since the hip flexors are unopposed by the effect of gravity on the distal leg.

    B **True**   the attachment of the glutei muscles to the greater trochanter achieves this and the proximal fragment is usually externally rotated.

    C **True**   this is due to the unopposed action of the adductor muscles. The hamstrings and quadriceps also produce some shortening of the leg.

    D **False**   extensive bleeding may occur particularly from the profunda vessels but the main artery and vein are not usually directly involved.

375 A **False**   transverse fractures are more common and usually produced by acute flexion of the knee. Direct injuries to the patella usually produce comminuted fractures.

    B **True**   the fragments may be held together by the capsule of the knee joint, although there is frequently a large haemarthrosis present which will require aspiration.

    C **False**   excision is only advisable in very severely comminuted fractures and even if this is necessary no prosthesis is required. Tendon suture provides quite good knee flexion.

    D **False**   provided the knee is maintained in extension, weight bearing can be readily undertaken. Active quadriceps exercise may be started on about the 10th day after the injury.

376 A **True**   these fractures are frequently compound. There is a relatively poor blood supply to the bones in this region, and interposition of muscle and superadded infection are frequent complications. Therefore the incidence of delayed union is high.

    B **True**   particularly if a twisting force is imparted to the foot.

    C **True**   the anterior surface of the tibia is unsupported by muscles and no splinting effect occurs.

    D **False**   these fractures are usually due to direct injury and are compound. Internal fixation is therefore best avoided.

377 A **False**   the ankle is more unstable in the inverted position.

    B **False**   this injury affects the lateral not the medial ligament of the joint.

    C **False**   nerve and vascular complications are exceedingly rare.

    D **True**   this injury requires external or internal fixation for 6 weeks prior to any weight bearing.

378   **Dislocation of the hip joint**
   A   is most common when the hip is in a neutral position
   B   is usually associated with a fracture of the acetabular rim
   C   usually results in the femoral head coming to lie anteriorly
        over the pubis or obturator externus
   D   may be associated with injuries of the sciatic nerve

379   **In fractures of the cervical spine**
   A   the odontoid process is usually damaged by extension
        injuries
   B   of the base of the odontoid process, the odontoid process is
        carried forward with the atlas
   C   non-union of the odontoid is uncommon
   D   involving a spinous process treatment is usually by internal
        fixation

378 A **False**   the most common dislocation is a posterior one and this is usually the result of force along the line of the femoral shaft when it is flexed at a right angle as in the sitting position. Thus, motorcyclists suffering a sudden deceleration frequently sustain posterior dislocations of the hip.

   B **True**   the posterior margin of the rim is most commonly affected.

   C **False**   this form of dislocation is occasionally seen but in the common posterior dislocation the head lies posterior to the acetabulum.

   D **True**   this serious, and sometimes permanent, disability sometimes complicates posterior dislocation of the hip.

379 A **False**   the commonest causes are flexion injuries such as occur in violent deceleration or from a blow to the back of the head.

   B **True**   it is maintained in this position by the transverse ligaments of the atlas.

   C **False**   the initial fracture may be painless and difficult to demonstrate but late films will show an area of sclerosis.

   D **False**   these, like fractures of a transverse process, are usually avulsion injuries and require no specific surgery. Active mobilisation should be encouraged once the initial pain has subsided.

18 Orthopaedic surgery

380 In rheumatoid arthritis
   A the principal lesion is an area of fibrinoid necrosis surrounded by fibroblasts
   B the synovial membrane characteristically undergoes marked hypertrophy
   C the fibrosis in the joint capsule and ligaments produces the main deforming forces in the early stages of the disease
   D the permanent deformity in the late stage of the disease is usually due to bone ankylosis

381 Rheumatoid arthritis
   A is characteristically symmetrical in its involvement of the more proximal joints
   B has an equivalent disease in childhood which is also associated with pericarditis
   C carries a worse prognosis if serological tests (such as the Rose Waller and Latex tests) are positive
   D Is characterised by the pes anserinus deformity

382 Acute osteomyelitis in childhood
   A is usually the result of compound bony injuries
   B is characterised by a constant bone pain
   C characteristically produces necrosis of the periosteum overlying the infected bone
   D is not demonstrable radiologically for the first 2 weeks of the disease

380 A **True**   these are the characteristic changes of the rheumatoid
            nodule.
    B **True**   this feature accounts for the joint swelling and the
            inflammatory mass which extends over the articular
            surface (known as the pannus).
    C **False** the early deformity is due to the laxity of the diseased
            capsule and ligaments together with associated
            muscle spasm.
    D **False** although bone ankylosis does occur it is rare. These
            permanent deformities are usually due to periarticular
            fibrosis.

381 A **True**   the disease starts distally and gradually extends to
            more proximal joints.
    B **True**   Still's disease — the childhood equivalent — is also
            characterised by skin rashes, lymphadenopathy and
            splenomegaly. The illness usually produces more
            systemic effects and is more rapid in onset than the
            adult form.
    C **True**   these tests are positive in approximately 25 per cent of
            cases.
    D **False** this term has no connection with rheumatoid arthritis
            (it in fact describes the division of the facial nerve).
            The proximal interphalangeal joints frequently show,
            however, a swan neck deformity produced by
            hyperextension of these joints.

382 A **False** it is usually haematogenous in origin, arising from
            foci such as boils, infected tonsils or urinary tract
            infections. Exogenous infections are more common in
            the adult form of the disease.
    B **True**   a constant pain of increasing severity is present from
            the earliest stages of the infection.
    C **False** bone necrosis frequently follows acute osteomyelitis.
            The dead bone is known as a sequestrum. The
            overlying periosteum usually survives and forms new
            subperiosteal bone known as the involucrum which
            thus often surrounds a subperiosteal abscess.
    D **True**   radiological evidence of bone infection may not be
            evident until the first subperiosteal new bone appears
            in 14 to 21 days. Antibiotic treatment must be
            instituted on clinical grounds as soon as the diagnosis
            is made.

226   Surgical MCQs

383   **In tuberculosis of the bone**
   A the local reaction is characterised by extensive new bone
      formation
   B the metaphysis of a long bone is the commonest site of
      involvement
   C the infection is usually secondary to a primary focus
      elsewhere in the body
   D extension of the bone abscess into a joint is common

384   **In osteoarthritis of the hip joint**
   A the articular cartilage undergoes initial hypertrophy and then
      becomes hardened and eburnated
   B the joint capsule becomes stretched and lax
   C the leg is usually adducted and externally rotated when the
      patient lies supine
   D a femoral osteotomy usually helps halt the progress of the
      disease process

385   **In Paget's disease of the bone**
   A the serum alkaline phosphatase is considerably raised
   B spiral fractures of the femur are common
   C deafness is a characteristic of the later stages of the disease
   D osteogenic sarcoma develops twice as commonly as in
      unaffected people

386   **Dyschondroplasia is characterised by**
   A a large skull with a short base and a snub nose
   B short stubby fingers (the trident hand)
   C being inherited as a Mendelian dominant
   D multiple enchondromata of the fingers and toes

383 A **False**   in bone tuberculosis, osteoporosis and bone lysis is usually present. There is much less tendency to new bone formation than in pyogenic bone infection.

    B **False**   the infection nearly always starts in the epiphysis.

    C **True**   it is a blood-borne metastatic infection which spreads from primary foci in the lungs, bowel or lymph nodes.

    D **True**   this is a consequence of the location of the infection and often results in joint destruction and extension of the abscess into the surrounding soft tissues. The abscesses show few of the classical signs of inflammation and may grow to a large size before presentation.

384 A **False**   the articular cartilage thins and becomes rough; the underlying bone then becomes dense and smooth (eburnated) and cysts usually develop in the perichondral bone.

    B **False**   the capsule becomes thick and fibrosed. At the extremes of movement some tearing may occur and this gives rise to further fibrosis.

    C **True**   some degree of fixed flexion deformity is also commonly present.

    D **True**   in some cases the joint changes are partly reversed. The operation should be performed before the head of the femur has collapsed. Improvement is unlikely if this has already occurred.

385 A **True**

    B **False**   though pathological fractures of the femur do occur in this condition, they are usually of the transverse variety and are typically in the subtrochanteric region of the femur

    C **True**   the bony thickening and deformity commonly involves the skull and may thus interfere with the transmission of sound vibrations. The spine, femur and tibia are the commonest sites of involvement.

    D **False**   there is a greatly increased rate of osteogenic sarcoma formation in these patients. It is more than 30 times that of the normal population and the tumour appears to be a particularly malignant variety.

386 A **False**   these are all features of achondroplasia — typified by

    B **False**   the short limbed circus dwarf. There is frequently a lordosis present.

    C **False**

    D **True**   the disease is also known as multiple enchondromatosis or Ollier's disease. It is due to the failure of ossification of areas of cartilage in the epiphyses. It is not familial.

387   Diaphysial aclasis is characterised by
   A   a defect in cartilagenous ossification
   B   multiple fractures and subsequent deformity
   C   blue sclera
   D   being familial in origin

388   Dupuytren's contracture of the palm
   A   is transmitted as a Mendelian dominant
   B   is predominantly seen in men
   C   has an association with glomerulonephritis
   D   which is long-standing, is often associated with secondary
       fibrosis of the interphalangeal joints

389   In a case of congenital dislocation of the hip
   A   there is a defect of the posterior rim of the acetabulum
   B   on bilateral hip abduction with the knees flexed there is often
       limited abduction on the diseased side
   C   reduction is sometimes hindered by a tight gluteus minimus
       muscle
   D   splinting of the limbs following reduction should be
       maintained until the femoral epiphysis returns to its normal
       density on X-ray examination

390   Slipped femoral epiphyses
   A   occur between the ages of 5 and 10 years
   B   typically are seen in overweight children
   C   are bilateral in 20 per cent of patients
   D   are displaced downwards and posterior in relation to the neck
       of the femur

387 A **True**   the condition is also known as multiple exostosis.
Large bony outgrowths appear at the ends of long
bones arising from the epiphyseal plate.
  B **False**   these features are typical of osteogenesis imperfecta
  C **False**   which often presents with frequent fractures following
trivial trauma at birth (as a stillbirth) or in later
childhood (osteogenesis imperfecta tarda).
  D **True**   and it is commoner in males.

388 A **False**   there is, however, an inherited predisposition to this
disease.
  B **True**   the frequency is 10:1.
  C **False**   it is associated with liver disease and chronic
alcoholism.
  D **True**   this may necessitate amputation of the digit.

389 A **False**   the acetabular defect is superior, although the
dislocation is always posterior. The consistency of this
defect is one of the factors supporting the genetic
theory of origin (20 per cent familial). Other theories
are abnormal intrauterine positioning and capsular
laxity due to maternal hormones.
  B **True**   this is the basis of Ortolani's test—the hip often
clicking (or jerking) into position to allow further
abduction.
  C **False**   characteristic causes limiting a closed reduction are a
tight psoas muscle, an hour-glass stricture of the
capsule, a thick ligamentum teres and an infolding of
the superior labrum glenoidale (known as the limbus).
  D **False**   reduction should be maintained until the acetabular
roof re-forms, which takes 6 to 9 months in those
cases diagnosed early.

390 A **False**   the age of peak incidence is 10 to 15 years.
  B **True**   boys are affected more commonly than girls.
  C **True**   carefull follow-up is therefore essential.
  D **True**   a lateral X-ray of the hip joint is therefore the most
informative.

391   Perthes disease of the hip
  A   is a degenerative disease of the elderly
  B   often presents with a fixed flexion deformity of the hip
  C   may, in most cases, be treated non-surgically
  D   has a better prognosis when diagnosed in a younger patient

392   Idiopathic scoliosis
  A   is the most common type of scoliosis
  B   usually appears between the ages of 10 and 12 years
  C   is more common in boys
  D   is sometimes familial

393   In benign tumours of cartilage
  A   chondromata and osteochondromata occur equally in the two sexes
  B   malignant changes occur in 10 per cent of cases of multiple osteochondromata
  C   chondromata usually occur in the epiphyses of long bones
  D   osteochondromata usually occur in the epiphyses of long bones

394   Chordomata
  A   of the base of the skull (spheno-occipital) develop in the remnants of Rathke's pouch
  B   of the sacrococcygial region develop in the remnants of the neural canal
  C   are characterised radiologically by central rarefaction of the bone and cortical thinning and expansion
  D   are commoner in females than in males

391 A **False**   this is a disease of young children particularly
between the ages of 5 and 10 years. Boys are affected
four times more frequently than girls. It is thought to
be due to an ischaemic necrosis of the epiphysis of the
head of the femur.

B **False**   the usual presentation is with pain in the hip and a
limp. X-rays may show fragmentation, flattening and
increased density of the femoral head.

C **True**   the deformity of the femoral head and thus the long-
term sequelae are minimised by non-weight-bearing
(often for more than one year).

D **True**   this is probably due to the smaller epiphysis in the
young child which has a better chance of being
revascularised.

392 A **True**   the scoliotic deformity produced is severe in this
group (the worst being due to the paralytic form).

B **True**   there often is marked deterioration over the following
years until the completion of vertebral growth.

C **False**   there is a predominance of this condition in girls. It

D **True**   has been suggested that the condition is due to
subclinical poliomyelitis but as the latter is equally
distributed in both sexes this appears unlikely. The
familial tendency may indicate a genetic aeticlogy.

393 A **True**   but the benign chondroblastoma is commoner in
males.

B **True**   but this is less common in solitary tumours and
occurs rarely in chondroblastomata.

C **False**   these tumours are usually present in the metaphysis
of long bones, particularly in the bones of the hands
and feet.

D **False**   these tumours are usually seen in the metaphysis of
long bones. Chondroblastomata occur primarily in the
epiphyses.

394 A **False**   these tumours develop from notochordal remnants
and usually occur at its cephalic or caudal extremity.

B **False**

C **False**   the characteristic radiological appearances are
progressive bone destruction and soft tissue swelling.

D **False**   they are twice as common in males and present
usually after the age of 30. The symptoms are mainly
due to neural involvement.

395   An osteoid osteoma
   A   usually presents in the adult
   B   is most frequently seen in the bones of the upper limb
   C   commonly presents with local pain
   D   demonstrates a small circular band of bony sclerosis
       surrounding a translucent area on X-rays

396   The osteoclastoma (giant cell tumour of bone)
   A   characteristically occurs in the shaft of a long bone
   B   is more common in females than males
   C   may be recognised by the subperiosteal new bone which
       overlies the tumour and is demonstrable radiologically
   D   is very rarely malignant

397   Osteogenic sarcomata
   A   are most frequent in the 10 to 25 year age group
   B   readily metastasise via the blood stream
   C   are frequently surrounded by non-malignant new bone
       formation
   D   when treated by conventional methods have a 50 per cent 5-
       year survival rate

395 A **False**   it most commonly present during adolescence.
     B **False**   any bone may be involved but there is a slight
                     predilection for the bones of the lower limb.
     C **True**   particularly so at night. Local tenderness also occurs.
     D **True**   these are the characteristic radiographic appearances
                     of osteoid osteoma and they may be confused with
                     those of a chronic pyogenic bone abscess.

396 A **False**   it is almost invariably situated at the end of a bone. It
                     can occur in any bone but is rare in flat bones.
     B **False**   it is twice as common in males and the commonest
                     age of presentation is in the third and fourth decades.
     C **False**   radiological characteristics do not include
                     subperiosteal new bone. There is cortical expansion
                     and thinning, together with rarefaction of the
                     underlying bone. The cortex may be totally destroyed
                     in the later stages of the disease.
     D **False**   local recurrence is present in almost half the cases
                     after attempted surgical removal and malignant
                     change is seen in about 15 per cent. Treatment should
                     be by wide excision.

397 A **True**   the majority occur in this age group, exceptions being
                     those occurring in late life in patients with Paget's
                     disease of the bone. Common sites are around the
                     knee and shoulder joint.
     B **True**   pulmonary metastases are particularly common.
                     Lymph node metastases are very uncommon.
     C **True**   the periosteum overlying an osteogenic sarcoma is
                     raised by the tumour. This produces the characteristic
                     radiological appearances of the overlying periosteum
                     having underneath it a triangular area of new bone
                     formation (Codman's triangle). The tumour itself
                     comprises radiating spicules of new bone formation
                     ('sunray') and variable degrees of lysis and sclerosis.
     D **False**   radical surgery is usually combined with preoperative
                     radiotherapy. Not more than 5 to 10 per cent of
                     patients survive 5 years. Recently there have been
                     encouraging reports of improved survival figures after
                     the use of multiple chemotherapy.

398   The Ewing's sarcoma of bone
    A is classically a disease of middle age and late years
    B can be effectively treated by radiotherapy
    C frequently results in a pathological fracture
    D usually occurs in the diaphyses of the long bones

399   Fibrosarcomata of the bone
    A are the most malignant of bone tumours
    B most commonly occur in the bones of the tarsus
    C demonstrate bone destruction with no new bone formation
        on X-ray
    D usually present with pulmonary metastases

400   Chondrosarcomata
    A which develop in the metaphysis are usually less well
        differentiated than those occurring around the epiphysis
    B quite commonly invade the neighbouring blood vessels
    C commonly metastasise to lymph nodes
    D characteristically present as a pathological fracture

398 A **False** the usual presentation is in infancy and up to the age of 25. It is more frequent in males.

B **False** survival varies from a few months to a few years. Whilst radiotherapy provides some symptomatic relief, neither this nor surgery is usually curative. The tumour is often multicentric in origin and adjuvant chemotherapy has been added to the treatment protocol with some encouraging improvement in the results.

C **False** the most frequent radiographic appearance is of overlapping layers of new subperiosteal bone formation, the so called 'onion peel' effect. This new bone has normal strength, thus pathological fractures are very uncommon.

D **True** it is extremely uncommon for any other portion of the bone to be affected.

399 A **False** they are slower growing than osteogenic sarcomata and a 5-year survival rate of approximately 25 per cent is frequently reported. Treatment is by radical amputation.

B **False** the sites of predilection are similar to those of the osteogenic sarcoma, i.e. in the ends of long bones, particularly the femur, tibia and humerus.

C **True** the absence of radiating bone spiculation distinguishes it from osteogenic sarcoma.

D **False** the most usual presentation is of a local, painful, progressive swelling around the knee, elbow or shoulder joint and sometimes a pathological fracture.

400 A **True** metaphyseal tumours often develop from osteochondromata whereas the peripheral tumours are formed of more mature cartilage. These tumours are slightly commoner in males and occur between the ages of 30 to 60 years.

B **True** extension into the blood vessels is quite frequent.

C **False** metastases are usually seen late in the disease and are blood-borne, commonly producing peripheral lung deposits. Lymph node metastases are rare.

D **False** the commonest presentation is of a painful bony swelling. Tenderness is present, particularly when haemorrhage and extraosseous extension has occurred.

19 Neurosurgery

401 Intracranial aneurysms
- **A** are the cause of the vast majority of cases of spontaneous subarachnoid haemorrhage
- **B** are multiple in 20 per cent of cases
- **C** frequently rebleed after an initial haemorrhage
- **D** which have ruptured require surgical treatment which involves clipping of the appropriate middle cerebral artery

402 In head injuries the causes of a rising intracranial pressure include
- **A** intracerebral haemorrhage.
- **B** cerebral oedema
- **C** rhinorrhoea
- **D** meningitis

403 In head injuries the signs of an expanding intracranial lesion include
- **A** a falling level of consciousness
- **B** a rising pulse rate
- **C** a falling blood pressure
- **D** small pupils

401 A **False**   intracranial aneurysms are the cause of over 50 per cent of spontaneous subarachnoid haemorrhage but the remainder are due to arteriovenous malformations, blood dyscrasias, antiocoagulant therapy and hypertension, together with a large group of unknown aetiology.

B **True**   these occur at arterial bifurcations around the circle of Willis.

C **True**   this carries with it a higher morbidity and mortality than the first bleed.

D **False**   surgical treatment where indicated is directed at (i) excluding the aneurysm by clipping it at its neck, (ii) reinforcing its walls with fascia or synthetic material, or (iii) promoting thrombosis by injecting into it or by reducing its blood flow, e.g. by a carotid ligation. Clipping of the middle cerebral artery will usually produce serious neurological complications.

402 A **True**   this is one of the three common types of post-traumatic intracranial haemorrhage. The others are considered in subsequent questions.

B **True**   this may develop within a few hours and contribute to the mortality of severe cases. It is normally treated by diuretic therapy, fluid restriction and steroids.

C **False**   this and ottorrhoea usually subside within a few days. If they persist, craniotomy and some form of surgical repair of the dura is undertaken. It is not directly related to increasing intracranial pressure.

D **True**   this may follow closed as well as open cerebral injuries but is it more common in the latter. Prophylactic antibacterial therapy is indicated in open injuries.

403 A **True**   this is the most important of signs. Ensure that reproducible factors (such as whether or not the patient knows his name, age and address and the manner in which he obeys simple commands) are fully recorded at frequent intervals.

B **False**   the reverse is the case, the pulse rate falls and the
C **False**   blood pressure rises These vital signs must be observed at least every 15 minutes until normal stable values are maintained.

D **False**   these may be present in the initial stage due to stimulation of the oculomotor nerve but progressive increase in pressure shifts the brain and puts pressure on the oculomotor nerves resulting in pupillary dilatation (small pupils are seen with pontine injuries and these carry a very bad prognosis).

404   Following head injuries surgical intervention is usually required for
   A   linear skull fractures
   B   cerebral oedema
   C   depressed skull fractures
   D   extradural haemorrhage

405   Head injuries may be complicated by
   A   hydrocephalus
   B   epilepsy
   C   diabetes insipidus
   D   diabetes mellitus

406   Chronic subdural haematomata
   A   are common in the young
   B   have a characteristic angiographic appearance
   C   should be treated surgically
   D   have a better postoperative prognosis than acute subdural haematomata

404 A **False**   linear skull fractures demand careful observation of
    B **False**   the patient's vital signs in order to detect such
complications as haemorrhage or infection. In the
absence of these signs they do not require surgery.
There is no satisfactory surgical cure for post-
traumatic cerebral oedema.

    C **True**   surgery is required in all but minor depressions over
non-vital areas.

    D **True**   this is usually due to damage of the middle meningeal
vessels often in association with linear fractures of the
temporal bone. Typically the patient loses
consciousness at the time of the accident due to
concussion. Consciousness then returns (the so called
lucid interval) until increasing intracranial pressure
results in a falling of the level of consciousness.
Emergency surgery is indicated to evacuate the clot
and control the haemorrhage.

405 A **True**   the advent of the CAT scan has revealed that post-
traumatic hydrocephalus may frequently follow
severe head injury. It is due to obstruction of the
aqueduct by blood and may require ventricular
drainage or an indwelling shunt.

    B **True**   the risks are highest in those who have had a post-
traumatic amnesia for more than 24 hours, dural
penetration, a missile injury or early epilepsy.

    C **True**   it is fortunately rare but follows pituitary necrosis
secondary to trauma or hypoxia.

    D **False**   this is not associated.

406 A **False**   they occur characteristically in the aged and often
follow quite minor injuries. They are rarely associated
with skull fractures.

    B **True**   the cortical vessels are displaced from the vault and
there is a shift in the midline structures away from the
side of the lesion. The CAT scan has now almost
completely replaced angiography as the primary
investigation.

    C **True**   Acute subdural haemorrhage follows severe trauma
    D **True**   and is often bilateral. It is associated with more severe
underlying permanent damage to the brain, and has a
worse prognosis than the chronic subdural
haematoma. The latter should be treated surgically
since it is generally associated with very minor
underlying cerebral injury and the results are good.

407 The characteristic signs of chronically raised intracranial pressure include
    A a bitemporal hemianopia
    B papilloedema
    C epilepsy
    D bradycardia

408 In a patient with a lumbar disc protrusion
    A loss of the knee jerk is characteristic of a second lumbar nerve root lesion
    B loss of dorsiflexion of the great toes indicates a third lumbar nerve root lesion
    C loss of sensation over the sole indicates a fourth lumbar nerve root lesion
    D loss of the ankle jerk indicates a first sacral root lesion

409 In lesions affecting the common peroneal (lateral popliteal) nerve
    A sensory loss is limited to the dorsal aspect of the first interdigital cleft
    B there is weakness of dorsiflexion of the foot
    C there is weakness of eversion of the foot
    D the toes become clawed

410 Brain abscesses
    A are usually secondary to sepsis elsewhere in the body
    B are frequently the consequence of throat infections
    C are usually multiple
    D should be treated by antibiotics without surgical drainage

407 A **False**   this characteristically follows pressure on the optic decussation from a pituitary tumour or a suprasellar meningioma.

    B **True**   papilloedema accompanies a raised intracranial pressure and is not, in its early phase, accompanied by visual symptoms.

    C **True**   this may be grand mal or focal in nature.

    D **True**   this is probably caused by the effect of pressure on the vasomotor centre. Other signs include a falling conscious level and a sixth nerve palsy.

408 A **False**   the knee jerk is mediated via the third and fourth lumbar nerve roots.

    B **False**   this useful physical sign indicates a lesion of the fifth lumbar nerve root.

    C **False**   the sole is supplied via the first sacral nerve root.

    D **True**

409 A **False**   this is the area of sensory loss associated with lesions of the anterior tibial nerve. Involvement of the common peroneal nerve gives rise to sensory loss over the lateral aspect of the leg and the dorsum of the foot.

    B **True**   the patient suffers from foot drop and walks with a

    C **True**   high stepping gait on the affected side.

    D **False**   this is seen in lesions of the tibial (medial popliteal) nerve due to paralysis of the intrinsic muscles of the foot.

410 A **True**   infection in the pleural or peritoneal cavity is the usual site of origin in the USA but infection

    B **False**   of the paronasal air spaces or chronic supporative otitis media are common causes in the UK.

    C **False**   since abscesses in the frontal or porietal lobes account for more than 50 per cent of brain abscesses. Multiple abscesses are rare and occur usually in immune suppressed patients.

    D **False**   Surgical drainage with appropriate antibiotic therapy is almost always required. It should be monitored by frequent CAT scans. In the few cases when diagnosis occurs at the stage of cerebritis with no pus success has followed CAT scan monitored antibiotic treatment.

411   Birth injuries involving the fifth and sixth cervical nerve roots of the brachial plexus
- A   are known as Klumpke's palsy
- B   are rarely followed by full recovery
- C   are characterised by the arm being held in the pronated and internally rotated position
- D   show weakness and wasting of the small muscles of the hand

412   Following a peripheral nerve injury
- A   loss of axon continuity is described as neuropraxia
- B   due to gunshot wounds primary nerve repair is desirable
- C   delayed suture is best performed one week after the injury
- D   delayed suture is best performed 3 months after the injury

413   After peripheral nerve section
- A   the axon grows distally at approximately 4 mm/day
- B   the growing end of the nerve can be localised by percussion
- C   primary nerve suture should usually be undertaken
- D   the motor endplates degenerate after 6 weeks and resuture after this period is rarely satisfactory

414   Brain tumours
- A   in the adult are most commonly glioblastomata multiforme
- B   in children are most commonly medulloblastomata
- C   of childhood are most commonly found in the posterior cranial fossa
- D   which arise extracerebrally are most commonly acoustic neuromata

411 A **False**   this injury is known as Erb's palsy. Klumpke's palsy is
                   a lesion involving the 8th cervical and 1st thoracic
                   roots of the brachial plexus and is a rare complication
                   of breech delivery.

   B **False**   full recovery is usual in this unjury. It is essential to
                   maintain passive movement and to splint the limb to
                   prevent contractions during the recovery phase
                   (recovery is unusual in Klumpke's palsy).

   C **True**   the limb is also adducted and splinting should
                   therefore maintain the limb abducted, externally
                   rotated and supinated.

   D **False**   this is characteristic of first thoracic nerve root injury.

412 A **False**   neuropraxia is temporary impairment of nerve
                   conduction. Loss of axon and nerve continuity are
                   described as axontmesis and neurotmesis
                   respectively.

   B **False**   primary nerve repair should only be considered in
                   uncontaminated wounds

   C **False**   the optimal time of nerve repair is 3 to 4 weeks after
   D **False**   the injury, providing there is no local infection and the
                   surrounding tissues have healed. The nerve ends can
                   then be mobilised, trimmed of new fibrous tissue and
                   carefully anastomosed.

413 A **False**   although this rate has been described in experimental
                   animals, in the clinical situation recovery rate is not
                   more than 1 to 1.5 mm/day.

   B **True**   this is known as Tinnel's sign and refers to the
                   paraesthesia produced over the growing nerve end in
                   response to slight trauma.

   C **False**   except in the rare instances of clean division (e.g.
                   accidental surgical division of the nerve) resuture is
                   best left for about 3 weeks when the damaged area is
                   clearly demarcated and local contamination has
                   subsided.

   D **False**   motor endplate degeneration takes a number of
                   months to occur.

414 A **True**   these are highly malignant showing rapid growth and
                   marked invasiveness.

   B **True**   these are by far the most common and together with
   C **True**   other posterior fossa tumours such as the cerebellar
                   astrocytoma make up the vast majority of childhood
                   intracranial tumours.

   D **False**   meningiomas are the commonest extracerebral
                   tumour followed by acoustic neuromas and pituitary
                   tumours.